PALEO DIET FOR BEGINNERS

Naturally Fight Diseases, Boost Energy and Improve Your Life

(Creating Your Paleo Lifestyle-delicious Recipes to Improve Your Health)

Martin Jones

Published by Tomas Edwards

Paleo Diet for Beginners: Naturally Fight Diseases, Boost Energy and Improve Your Life (Creating Your Paleo Lifestyle-delicious Recipes to Improve Your Health)

ISBN 978-1-989744-66-6

All rights reserved. No part of this guide may be reproduced in any form without permission in writing from the publisher except in the case of brief quotations embodied in critical articles or reviews.

Table of contents

Part 1

Introduction -What is the Paleo Diet?

Over the last 2 and half millennia, the primitive human being scourged as well as poked around for meat, vegetables, sea-food, roots, fruits and nuts. This stage of history in which man had to hunt for his food and there was no concept of growing his own food, it is called the Paleolithic age. People actually had to go out in the open wild and manage their food. Back in that time certainly "picking this or that" was not an available option.

Other names for the Paleo dietary regime are

☐   The Primal Diet

☐   The Stone Age dietary regime,

☐   The hunter-gathering dietary regime

☐   The caveman dietary regime

The names are them-selves explaining what resources they used to have in that age, during the Stone Age, people had to use "stones" as a weapon to hunt for food. They ate raw and sometimes burnt food in open flames. The hunter gathering dietary regime name suggests that people learnt to hunt animals during that period, be it a wild bird, a fish from the sea or a goose. And the name "caveman dietary regime" came into being because during the Stone Age people used to live in caves.

Over the countless years, we have evolved so much but some things are same for us as they were for our forefathers of prehistoric era. The concept of growing own food (farming) was introduced some 10'000 years ago. In these years, our alimentary system had only evolved a little bit.

Now this system of eating is commonly known as PALEO, the new concept of this diet bases on principle of "healthy diet".

With evolution, we may have advanced in terms of knowledge and physical characteristic but our body still yearns for the "Healthy diet" AKA paleo diet. In modern medicine, the Paleo diet was introduced for the first time in 1970s by Walter L. Voegtlin, a famous Gastroenterologist.

In his publication (called the Stone Age Diet) he elaborated that humans were carnivores and their basic food requirements included proteins, fats and carbohydrates for the normal functioning of their systems.

It is quite evident that we all strife for a good health, that is why the proverb, "health is wealth" came into being. If we look at a simple graph, we can detect that obesity has become a worldwide problem in the last 3 decades.

The diets of our era are enriched with refined sugars, fried edibles and preserving substances (all a rich source of carbohydrates). In the light of emerging health issues of our times, the concept of Paleo diet is being reviewed with new interest for finding solutions to our problems. Of course to lead a healthy and productive life we need a good amount of carbohydrates every day.

But this does not mean that we should let go of ourselves and engulf as much fried food as we possibly can! There is a right way to do everything and the right healthy way of incorporating carbohydrate in our everyday meal, PALEO diet has done a phenomenal job.

Advantages Of Paleo Diet

The benefits of the Paleo Diet have been extensively investigated and established in many intellectual publications. It is astounding to note that by just alternating our foods, we can bring notable changes in our lives, overall leading to improvement in the quality.

It does not can a toll on your everyday routine to blend this diet in, in fact if you actually follow the diet, thing may just get much easier.

At the beginning, everything we start seems a bit tough and often times you feel you cannot handle it. But the idea is to look at the permanent preservation and be steady in your goal. Isn't it much easier to be able to work all day long and still be able to play with your 3 year old after getting home?

It does not matter in which stage or age you are in, Paleo does not require you to be super old, anyone can try this and no matter how young or old you are, you can be benefitted by it. Check out how you can get benefitted by this diet.

Here are some effects of Paleo diet on our daily lives.

Fat loss: The Paleo way of life offers an exceptional diet. One can quench the thirst of one's taste buds while at the same time; he is able to burn his excessive fats. Paleo diet is low in carbohydrates, rich in proteins. Carbohydrates are the primary energy source for the body. When carbohydrates are not included in diet, the body relies on burning stored fats to release energy. All the veggies that are super important to lose weight are included in the Paleo diet.

VEGGIES THAT CAN HELP YOU LOSE WEIGHT

Vegetables play a big role in our meal. They are added in the diet in the form of salad, soup, or as whole meal itself. They are the natural resources and hence, they are beneficiary to our body and mind. There are varieties of vegetables available in the nature and everybody possess their different functions and here we are going to discuss about some vegetables which actually can cause weight loss and fat burn and these are listed as follows:

☐   <u>Green leafy vegetables:</u> Spinach, cabbage, broccoli, lettuce, cauliflower, are some of the examples of green leafy vegetables. They are the best sources of folic acid and other trace elements which are essential for normal nerve functioning. They prevent certain heart diseases and catalyze the normal cell growth. These all vegetables cut off calories in one or another way.

☐ **Cauliflower:** Cauliflower is a great source of vitamin C, folic acid and phytonutrients that can fight with cancer.

☐ **Lettuce:** Lettuce is high on the list of diet friendly food and it contains merely 60-70 calories per pound and it is a rich source of vitamin B, folic acid, manganese, which further helps in regulating blood sugar level and immunity.

☐ **Spinach:** Spinach consists mainly of iron, folic acid, vitamin K &C, antioxidants, beta carotene. It also possesses lutein which protects our eyes from macular degeneration caused by ageing. It can be taken in the form of salad with other vegetables.

☐ **Root vegetables:** Root vegetables such as carrots, radish, parsnips, sweet potatoes are rich sources of fiber and the food items which possess fiber pass out the digestive system faster than other foods. Some nutritionists recommend eating eighteen grams of fiber per day.

☐ **Carrots:** Carrots are rich in water content and its juice will pile up more fiber in your body and can keep your hunger on hold for few hours. Also, they possess fewer calories as compared to other foods such as pasta.

☐ **Radish:** These vegetables are rich in potassium, folic acid, antioxidants, and sulfur compounds and these elements enhance the digestion. The leafy part consists mainly of vitamin C and calcium as compare to the root part.

☐   Sweet potato: This vegetable is enriched with vitamin A and few grams of fiber which means that you can eat them to fulfill your daily requirement and on other side you can also lose some calories. It possesses half of the calories as compare to other variety of potato.

☐   Kale: kale is a great source of beta carotene, vitamin C and isothiocyanates (photochemical), and these three boosts up the detoxifying mechanism in the body by catalyzing their respective enzymes. It is considered good for reducing or cutting some of your calories. It can be served in form of soups also and in several studies it's been proven that soups provide a great satiety which means that you can feel full on having fewer calories.

☐   Brussels: These are one of the sweet vegetables which possess very low calories (28) and high amount of fiber (2 grams). They also possess isothiocyanates just like kale. Vitamin A, C &K are also one of its constituents.

Paleo diet also includes leaving the "bad drinks" out and including a lot of good drinks such as water, coconut milk, tea, vegetable juice and fruit juice etc. They work tremendously well to lose weight.

☐   Water: Water is a natural beverage and it is healthy for our body in all aspects. Water is on the top as compare to all the beverages and it is also a good choice for an effective weight loss.

Make water your go-to beverage choice and if you can't take plain water as it is; then make a blend in its taste by adding slice of lemon, lime, cucumber or tomato into it.

Consumption of water containing fruits and vegetables are another source of providing great amount of water to the body. In recent studies, it's been proven that women who consume high water content foods show decreased body weight and smaller waistlines.

The reason for this is the increased satiety caused by the consumption of these foods.

☐ Vegetable juice: Vegetable juice is a great source of fiber and nutrients which helps you in healthy way of losing weight. You can get them canned or homemade also but fresh juice is considered healthier than canned juice. Low sodium containing juice proves to be of more benefit than the others. It can keep your satisfied for few hours and the tangy taste also keep your taste buds happy.

☐ Another method of taking vegetable is vegetable soup; it is a nutritious and warm way of providing great health and weight loss to your body as it includes fibers and other nutritious substances. It's been proven that the person who starts his/her meal with vegetable soup eat 20 percent less calories over the course of their meal.

☐ Tea: Green tea boosts up the metabolism of the body and in this way it enhances weight loss. Green tea should be tried hot or iced with a little bit of honey or low sugar level. In addition to green tea, there are also other varieties of tea such as oolong teas and black teas, which are filled with antioxidants and which can remove toxins from the body.

☐ Coconut Milk: Milk is an excellent source of vitamin D, protein, and calcium which helps in building up the musculoskeletal system of our body. For losing weight, you need to opt out skim milk which is free of cream with retaining other nutrients in it. One can also have almond milk or cashew milk too. They have the same effect.

It's been proven in a large study that women who are light to moderate drinkers have less chances of gaining weight than those who don't drink at all.

Live Healthy: The paleo dietary plans offer a protection against several lethal diseases. You can actually get cured from diseases like diabetes mellitus, hypertension, cerebrovascular accidents, and carcinomas of GI tract, ischemic heart disease and Alzheimer's disease.

While you can still be in your prescribed medicine, Paleo diet does not guarantee you that you would get cured 100% by it, but it does ease up your metabolism and helps you increase antibody power.

Tonic for digestive system: Paleo diet can actually work wonders if you have digestion problems. When you have a digestion problem, we know everything comes at a stop, and you cannot enjoy anything, all you want is some ease.

Paleo diet acts as a tonic for digestive system. A number of digestive problems such as inflammatory bowel disease (crohn disease and ulcerative colitis), IBS and constipation can be prevented by being in paleo diet.

Protection against Acne: Now the problem of acne is something that is troubling teenagers worldwide, especially women seems to be more alarmed by it.

We try and do everything we possibly can to make sure our skin is flawless, because no matter what makeup you use, if your skin is full of acne, it doesn't help! Normal diet causes sudden release of insulin in the body because of its extended carbohydrate content. This insulin causes sebaceous glands to secrete thick viscous sebum which gets lodged in the ducts of glands causing blockage.

This leads to formation of acne.

The Paleo diet doesn't have this effect on us. The insulin release is regular and sebum retains its normal consistency. Now if only eating 'good food' can get rid of the awful scars on the face, why wouldn't one try it!

Live longer: The caveman's diet is rich in anti-oxidant substances. They slow down cellular breakdown, improves their functioning and all of these effects in combination prolong life.

The basic cause of death in living beings is loss of cellular functioning which causes organ systems to shut down. And the person dies.

Good Skin: Paleo diet contains a lot of antioxidant, which is very good for the skin. So Paleo diet can help you get you a very healthy and beautiful skin. Also as the Paleo diet endorses a continuous usage of different fruits and vegetables, the diet has a good amount of Vitamin C. We all know vitamin C is extremely good for the skin.

Say bye to lethargic Feelings: Paleo diet can also help you combat with lethargic feelings. We all know how nerve wrecking it is to have piles of work on your desk but no amount of energy in you to get up and do the work. Only when you eat something very heavy and unhealthy, you get that lethargic feeling. You can have heavy meal

Basic Concept Of Paleo Diet

Paleo diet is very easy to follow. There are misconceptions that it is costly than ordinary diet. As a matter of fact, it is much cheaper not only in the short term but also in the long term.

For the sake of diet, 60-65% of the recommended daily allowance should be of animal origin (meat etc); up to 35% should come from plants. The proteins should make the bulk of diet (usually the animal origin food is rich in proteins). The carbohydrates should range between 35-40% of RDA.

What Makes Up A Normal Meal In

Paleo Diet?

Paleo diet is just like expeditions. With each step, with each bite, you experience something new. You have the option of making your own food. Make your own new combinations every time you eat. Let your taste buds experience new tastes.

Don't just settle from fast food or other junk foods available. Have a meal that is not only delicious but also nutritious, healthy and life-prolonging.

Below is a brief itinerary of food items should be an integral part of your daily diet.

PROTIENS

Meat	Game	Poultry	Fish	Shellfish	Eggs
Beef	Pheasant	Goose	Tuna	Lobster	Chicken eggs
Veal	Deer	Chicken	Salmon	Shrimp	Goose eggs
Pork	Duck	Turkey	Trout	Scallops	Duck eggs
Lamb	Wild Turkey	Quail	Halibut	Crab	Quail eggs
Goat	Rabbit	Duck	Sole	Clams	
Rabbit	Moose		Bass	Mussels	
Sheep	Woodcock		Haddock	Oysters	
Wild Boar	Elk		Turbot		
Bison			Cod		

Tilapia
Walleye
Flatfish
Grouper
Mackerel
Herring
Anchovy

VEGETABLES

Standards	Green Leafy	Squash	Root	Mushrooms
Cauliflower	Collard Greens	Butternut	Turnips	Oyster
Broccoli	Lettuce	Spaghetti	Carrots	Button
Celery	Spinach	Acorn	Beets	Portabella
Bell Peppers	Watercress	Pumpkin	Parsnips	Chanterelle
Onions	Beet Top	Zucchini	Artichokes	Porcini
Leeks	Dandelion	Yellow Summer	Rutabaga	Shiitake
Green Onions	Swiss Chard	Buttercup	Sweet Potatoes	Criminal
Eggplant	Mustard Greens	Crookneck	Radish	Morel
Brussels	Kale		Yams	

Sprout			
Artichokes	Turnip Greens		Cassava
Asparagus	Seaweed		
Cucumber	Endive		
Cabbage	Arugula		
Okra			
Avocados			

SUPPORTING PLAYERS

Fats	Fruits	Nuts & Seeds	Flavor Enhancers	Fresh & Dry Herbs
Olive Oil	Apples	Brazil Nuts	Cayenne Pepper	Parsley
Avocado	Oranges	Pistachios	Chilies	Thyme
Coconut Oil	Bananas	Sunflower Seeds	Ginger	Lavender
Clarified Butter	Strawberry	Pumpkin Seeds	Onions	Mint
Lard	Cranberry	Sesame Seeds	Garlic	Rosemary
Tallow	Grapefruit	Pecans	Black Pepper	Chives

Veal Fat	Peaches	Walnuts	Hot Peppers	Tarragon
Duck Fat	Pears	Macadamia Nuts	Star Anise	Oregano
Coconut Flesh	Nectarines	Pine Nuts	Mustard Seeds	Dill
Nut Oils	Plums	Chestnuts	Fennel Seeds	Bay Leaves
Nut Butter	Pomegranates	Cashews	Cumin	Sage
Lamb Fat	Pineapple	Hazelnuts	Turmeric	Coriander
	Grapes	Almonds	Cinnamon	
	Papaya		Paprika	
	Cantaloupe		Nutmeg	
	Kiwi		Cloves	
	Lychee		Vanilla	

Foods That You Should Avoid

As it is evident that the list is rather long and one can even pick from this broad list which ones they would incorporate in their everyday lives and which ones they would leave out, there are certain foods that you MUST leave out of your diet. The foods that you should refrain from are refined carbohydrates.

They are obtained from processed foods (e.g. sugar, bread etc). These foods are deadly to the human body. Our digestive system is not made to digest these foods.

The breakdown products of these substances accumulate in body and ultimately cause lethal disease by causing cellular breakdown. These foods have become everyday part of our diet because they are so easy to get.

Every restaurant has abundance of these substances. By going through extensive refining, the grains, cereals and other of such foods lose their real importance for humans.

They now only serve to fill the stomach. But we must not go by the taste alone, we must think about the permanent impact those food would have in our body later on.

This does not mean Paleo food are not tasty, in fact they can be equally delicious if cooked a little tactfully.

Tips for the Paleo Lifestyle

The foods that are available these days have practically no nutritious value as compare to Paleo diet. We have moved so far away from the nature that eating real food that we have to hunt and kill first seems very odd.

☐ Be meticulous: An organized mind saves times. Be prepared, have stores of Paleo food in your home. Because when you have Paleo foods at hand, in your refrigerator, you won't have to go out to buy anything.

☐ Plan Your Meals: Now that you have foods in your refrigerator, the next step is planning your meals. You should make a mixture of foods for your meals. In this way, not only you will experience new taste every time but you will be more attracted ton this way of life.

☐ Where to shop: Change your shop. Don't shop at superstores any more. Find organic food stores. Find the farmers, butchers and fresh vegetable stores in your area. You should always have a list of things on you when you go for shopping. This list should be organized. Hunt for fresh food. Don't choose packed goods. Initially, you might find it tiring but with the passage of time, you will get used to it.

☐ Clean Your kitchen store: Rid yourself of processed food in your home. If you find it hard to part from them, just remember that they are the killers. Clean the pantry and be ready to welcome the paleo lifestyle with open arms.

☐ Know your stove: The processed foods can be obtained as pre-cooked foods. This is not satisfying as you can't mold them to their own needs. The processed foods have carbohydrates as their basic component.

In Paleo diet, there is a wide variety of food that is there for you to eat. Cooking your own food is the best possible way to take maximum benefit from your food. You have spent your hard earned money on food. You deserve the best. You will never get tired of your food.

☐ Make your own food dressings: The food dressings available on the market are not naturally prepared and they are also full of preservatives (which are harmful to your health). However, there is no Most of the condiments on the taste of food without dressing. And you will find them way more appetizing than those available commercially. And they will be cheaper to make.

☐ Regular Exercise: Just altering your eating behavior will cause a natural weight loss. This will take some time. But if you want rapid weight loss, start exercising regularly and you will notice a big difference in yourself.

You will fell more energetic, full of life and your speed of response will increase many folds. Your mind will sharpen, your stamina will increase and you will look younger for your years.

☐ Find People like yourself: in the beginning, you might find it difficult to follow Paleo diet. Your steps might falter as this way is hard and road is long. If you are serious and you want to have long term benefits, find people like yourself. Joining a group will strengthen your convictions. It will also allow you to share ideas with your peers.

Gone are the days where one actually had to eat only steamed up vegetables in their diet. Surely if you eat steamed vegetable 3 times a day, diet would be horrible thing to adopt. Paleo diet does not make you feel like you are on a diet, the food tastes great and it works miraculously on your body.

Paleo Diet Concerns

While starting a Paleo diet, one is always worried or rather concerned about their dessert because it is obvious dessert demands unnatural sweetening, so the ultimate question is whether or not desserts can be made without having unnatural sweetening?

Luckily nutritionists and dietitians have come up with amazing recipes that does not involve unnatural sweetening. To have sweetness in your dessert, you need to add raw honey to it.

In addition, Paleo desserts that needs diary can easily be substituted with milk from coconut, almond and cashew etc. Also the flours can be substituted with almond flour, coconut flour etc.

Paleo Diet Recipes

Chicken Kofta on Ramen Noodles

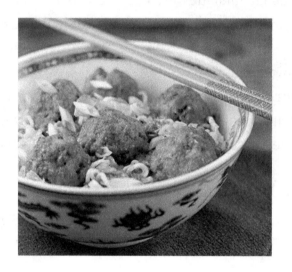

Servings: 2

PREPARATION TIME: 10 minutes

COOKING TIME: 30 min

Ingredients:

- ☐ 2 chicken breasts cut into small pieces

- ☐ ½ cup of wheat flour

- ☐ 2 tbsp of rice flour

- ☐   1 egg

- ☐ 4 tbsp of olive oil

- ☐ 1 tsp of paprika
- ☐ 1 tsp of turmeric
- ☐ 1 tsp of garam-masala
- ☐ 4 scallions, chopped
- ☐ 2 bell pepper, chopped
- ☐ A pinch of sea salt
- ☐ 1 pack of ramen noodle

Direction:

1. In a pan, boil the ramen noodle, drain, and set aside for now.

2. In a blender, add the chicken, chilies, scallions. Blend well until the chicken is well incorporated.

3. Season it with salt and spices.

4. Combine the chicken mixture with flours.

5. In another saucepan, heat the olive oil and deep fry the chicken balls.

6. Now put the chicken balls on top of ramen noodles.

7. Sprinkle some chopped scallions on top.

Creamy Chicken Curry

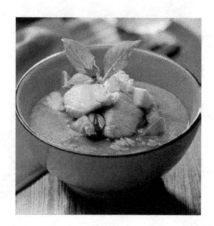

Servings: 6

PREPARATION TIME: 20 minutes

COOKING TIME: 3 hours

Ingredients:

- ☐ 1 pound of chicken, cut into little pieces

- ☐ 6 tbsp of raw honey

- ☐ 1 cup of coconut milk

- ☐ 1 tsp of cashew paste

- ☐ 1 tsp of chopped mint

- ☐ 3 tbsp of chicken broth

- ☐ Salt to taste

- ☐ Pepper to taste

- ☐ 3 tbsp of olive oil

Direction:

1. In a crockpot, heat the oil and fry the chicken for 5 min

2. Add the spices and cashew paste

3. Stir for another 5 min and pour in the coconut milk

4. Stir and pour in the broth

5. Add the honey

6. Add the mint and cook for 3 hours

Juicy Collard leaves surprise

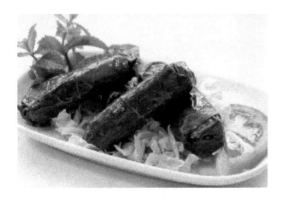

Servings: 4

PREPARATION TIME: 10 minutes

COOKING TIME: 30 min

Ingredients:

☐   A handful of collard leaves

☐   1/2 pound of shrimp

- ☐ 2 tbsp of cashew butter
- ☐ 4 tbsp of olive oil
- ☐ 4 onions, chopped
- ☐ 3 chillies, chopped
- ☐ 4 red tomatoes,
- ☐ 1 medium size cabbage
- ☐ ½ cup of walnuts
- ☐ 1 tsp of lime juice
- ☐ 2 tbsp of honey
- ☐ 1 tsp of cumin powder
- ☐ 1 tsp of black pepper
- ☐ Salt to taste

Direction:

1. Chop the shrimps. Slice up the tomatoes, and the cabbage.

2. In a saucepan, heat the butter

3. Fry the onions, chilies, veggies, nuts.

4. Season with salt and all the other spices.

5. Stir in the chopped shrimp.

6. Add the lime juice and stir. Drizzle the honey on top.

7. Stir for nearly 10 min and set aside.

8. Now place the collard leaves on top of a plain surface, fill the middle with the shrimp mixture.

9. Roll up the collard leaves tightly. Again heat the olive oil and fry the collard wraps. Sprinkle some salt and pepper on top. Serve hot.

Juicy Salmon Fry in Honey

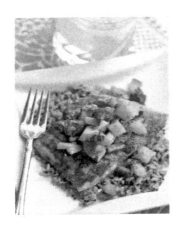

Servings: 2

PREPARATION TIME: 10 minutes

COOKING TIME: 30 min

Ingredients:
- ☐ ½ pound of salmon, deboned

- ☐ 4 tbsp of honey

- ☐ 1 tsp of red chili paste

- ☐ 1 tsp of ginger garlic paste

- ☐ 1 tsp of cumin

- ☐ 1 tsp of black pepper

- ☐ Fresh coriander, chopped

- ☐ 2 tbsp of cashew butter

- ☐ ½ cup of ripe mangoes, cut into small pieces

- ☐ Steamed brown rice

- ☐ Salt to taste

Direction:

1. Marinate the salmon with the chili paste, ginger garlic paste, honey and salt and pepper.

2. Refrigerate for 2 hours.

3. In a saucepan, heat the butter

4. Golden fry the salmon from both sides.

5. Plate the salmons on top of the brown rice.

6. Garnish with fresh coriander, and ripe mangoes.

10 Frequently Asked Questions about

Paleo Diet

Below are the most common questions people ask regarding Paleo diet.

Question 1: What is Paleo diet?

Answer: Paleo diet is a diet that helps you be healthy without being too keen on what you're eating as long as you leave out some of the heavy carbohydrate food, and sugar, and flour, dairy. It is also known as "Caveman Diet", "Primal Diet", "stone age diet" etc because research have shown that our ancestors of that era used to eat in this way.

Question 2: How costly is Paleo Diet?

Answer: Paleo diet is not at all costly, in fact you cannot even associate the term of "budgeting" with this diet as it doesn't require any extra money. It may help you save some bucks as well since the requirement of meat in this diet is rather less. Anyone can try this without worrying about the budget.

Question 3: What to eat and not to eat in a Paleo diet?

Answer: The list of what one can eat in Paleo diet is rather long, however; to sum it up short, one can have all the fruits and veggies that are low in carbohydrate. One can eat dairy such as coconut milk, butter etc. One can have chicken, beef, pork, shrimp, tilapia, crab, oysters, lamb, turkey, bacon, eggs etc.

Now for the non-eating part, one cannot eat grains such as wheat, oat, rye etc. Legumes like pinto beans, soy beans, kidney beans, navy beans etc. Nuts such as peanuts are off the limit.

Question 4: Can paleo diet other than making you healthy, help you lose weight?

Answer: Absolutely yes. Paleo diet contains the type of ingredients that help you gain energy, fastens your metabolism and gives your enough protein that you need, but since it cuts back in the carbohydrate, the body burns its existing fat, hence you lose weight automatically.

Question 5: What are the benefits of following this paleo diet?

Answer: There are several benefits. You can get reduce weight in the most natural way. You can flight back several diseases. You can live a healthier life for the longest time. You can kiss acne goodbye. You can get flawless healthy skin. The list goes on.

Question 6: Does recipes get compromised if you are in a paleo diet?

Answer: This is a common notion amongst most people that are thinking of trying Paleo diet but refrain from it thinking it would be impossible for them to find good recipes. There is no such compromised involve in the diet.

One can enjoy all sorts of good food; they can have varieties in their breakfast, have lunch that includes other recipes than salads, and have desserts just like other people. The idea is

28

that some ingredients would be substituted with other healthy ingredients.

Question 7: What makes Paleo Diet different from the other famous diets?

Answer: Paleo diet is in a way superior to any other diet because it does not cover only one thing at a time, for instance, any other FAD diet would focus solely on losing weight or reaching a certain level. Sometime the goal is to fight a disease.

But the interesting thing is all of these diet stops after a point, after reaching a point, the diets ceases to continue. As it turns out you tend to get back to your previous shape after a point.

On the other hand, Paleo diet helps you lose weight, set your hormonal balance correct, gets your metabolism set in the right motion. It makes your body fit and helps your gene expression be positive. Helps you be athletic and healthy.

Question 8: Paleo has bacon and egg in the diet, how can those be healthy?

Answer: Who does not love good bacon in the morning, with your fried or poached eggs on the side, your broccoli with salt and pepper and your favorite fruit be it strawberry or kiwi. If you have to leave out bacon from the diet, certainly it would not be much fun.

Egg and bacon both comes respectively from chicken and pig that are fed pure organic food, hence both are very nutritious food. It is no surprise that eggs are full of protein and nutrition, so it bacon.

Question 9: Is Paleo diet like a FAD diet?

Answer: A FAD diet usually concentrates on losing weight alone, once that goal is achieved; the diet requires you to stop. Paleo does help you lose weight in the process, but it doesn't solely focus on losing weight, it focuses on a healthy living in general.

It is not that you can start and stop because the end result has been achieved. It is not a seasonal thing or a onetime thing rather it is an all-time healthy living diet that eases up all your petty issues in addition.

Question 10: Can I still maintain my diet even when I eat outside occasionally?

Answer: We often eat outside in different occasions and sometimes in different parties, the question remains whether we can stay in that Paleo diet even when we are eating outside. There is no hard and fast rulebook on how you can continue your diet in that condition.

It solely depends on you, because at end of the day you would have to decide which road you would like to go by, if you know you need to stick to your diet then you would pick the food that are on your diet list. Having Paleo friendly food on any menu is not that hard because they are all very easy to get ingredients.

Also if you do not have any health condition and you know that eating something out of your diet chart would not cause you too much problem, then in such occasion you may just cut yourself some slack and dig in.

Question 11: Should I stop my Paleo diet when I lose all my extra weight?

Answer: First and foremost Paleo diet is not a weight loss project and it does not focus on weight losing alone. However; if you do try this diet for losing weight, it would definitely help you lose weight, but once you lose all that extra fat, it is not encouraged to stop.

The reason is simple, if you continue with Paleo; you can be on the healthier side, be a fit person, fight back diseases and have a very simple and healthy eating manner.

Question 12: If we do not eat enough carbohydrate, don't we be unhealthy?

Answer: Paleo diet requires you to consume a lot of protein and cuts back on the carbohydrate because usually carbohydrate is what gets stuck in your body and causes obesity.

But consuming too much protein helps you to burns your existing fat in your body and uses that carb to give you energy. Also this is a noteworthy point that you do not eat too much protein while being in a Paleo diet, rather you just eat enough.

So eating protein does not make you unhealthy in any way rather it helps you lose weight.

Question 13: What would be a Paleo diet meal (breakfast/ lunch/ dinner) is like?

Answer: For the breakfast, you can have the traditional egg in any way you want, be it poached, scrambled or boiled or even fried. Have your bacon with broccoli on the side, season with salt and pepper. Also a good fruit or vegetable juice would be good.

For the lunch, a very healthy and delicious salad would do, alongside the salad, have grilled chicken or salmon. Have some strawberries or blueberries on the side. Also have your favorite dipping sauce on the side, the dipping sauce should of course be made out of Paleo diet recipes.

For the afternoon, if your stomach starts reasoning with you, have smoked or grilled nuts (almond, macadamia, walnut etc). Also try the yummy coconut milk or almond milk.

For the dinner, have roasted beef or lamb (they must be grass-fed). Have roasted carrots or beet roots or Brussels sprout on the side.

Question 14: Caveman died very young, so eating like them wouldn't increase our chance of dying early?

Answer: This is purely a myth that 'caveman died very early'. Even though there was no data that could prove this hypothesis, but everyone believed this myth because they didn't know any better.

The notion evolved because during Paleolithic age, children and young people died at an alarming rate. But they died because they didn't have enough food, enough protection against wild animals and against the Mother Nature itself. Also life expectancy back then was around 39 and in a very later point it moved to 54.

Only in the last century the life expectancy suddenly grew broader.

Question 15:Isn't it advised by doctors that 'too much saturated fat is bad' and one should rather stick to whole grains?

Answer: Doctors know the very basic of nutrition and their field of study does not require them to go further in that. Also doctors focus on treating a problem rather than prevent the problem.

Which means you cannot expect a cure until you are affected by any disease, but Paleo diet does not wait for you to get affected, it put forth a plan that can help you before you face your problem.

The doctors that are more aware of nutrition and studies further would cohesively tell you to start Paleo diet. Few of the doctors already have taken initiative to side with Paleo and spread awareness.

CONCLUSION

The Paleo Diet is proven to shed pounds and have a healthier life. Add exercise to the mix and you can achieve the lean, sexy bodies seen on fitness models.

Despite popular belief, the Paleo lifestyle is not restrictive and can actually open your palette to a whole new world of culinary experiences.

There are a variety of high quality cookbooks and website that will help you along the way. Once you experience the transformation you will wonder how you ever functioned. Get the most of your life and enjoy optimum fitness with the Paleo diet plan.

Part 2

Introduction

This book contains proven steps and strategies on how to rapidly lose weight by following the paleo diet.

And if you follow the guidelines presented herein, I do not doubt in my mind that you will be able to succeed 60 Day Paleo Challenge as well. The recipes and bits of advice found in this book serve to guide you in a direction that leads to improved overall health and stamina. It is not about starving yourself, or counting carbs; the 60-Day Paleo Challenge is more than a diet or any other kind of food regimen. The 60-Day Paleo Challenge is a distinct way of life. Thank you for reading!

Delicious recipes that nourish the body and soul. Foods that are clean, pure, and perfect for staying in shape. Methods that encourage weight loss fill you up for hours at a time and make you feel better and more energetic. These are all positive aspects of the paleo diet. By eating healthy, unprocessed foods, the way they were intended, you will lose weight, feel more robust, and have more energy. It is one of the healthiest ways to eat.

Thanks again for downloading this book, I hope you enjoy it!

Chapter 1: What is a Paleo Diet?

The Paleolithic lifestyle as a dietary concept was initially endorsed by Dr. Walter Voegtlin. His book, <u>The Stone Age Diet</u>, was printed in 1975 and paved the way for some several Paleolithic advances, all similar in their core beliefs but with a variety of regulations and limitations.

The Paleolithic period was pre-agricultural for the majority of the time, and particular foods that we eat in great quantity now were incongruous for Paleolithic humans to use in their unprocessed form. A technique of consuming that goes back to fundamentals; Paleolithic diets are about consuming food the way our predecessors did.

The Paleo diet is primarily focused almost selectively on authentic, unprocessed foods that have been prevalent for thousands of years.

Eating in this approach eliminates the additives, salt, and sugars that are time and again included in highly processed foods. So, whether you like it or not, by progressing from consuming processed foods to actual, whole grains, it is practically unfeasible <u>not</u> to make improved eating choices and start feeling healthier.

Paleo diet followers intend to eat as organically as possible, going for grass-fed meats, plenty of fruit and vegetables, and natural foods, such as nuts and seeds. Some lenient adaptations of the regimen permit prohibited foods that were not accessible during Paleolithic times, like low-fat dairy goods and yams, while some followers even go as far as strictly avoiding fruit and vegetables considered to contain a higher level of fructose.

Many Paleo diet supporters consider our digestive systems have undergone very little modification ever since, and for that reason foods such as some of the ones listed below induce unnecessary pressure on the gastrointestinal tract:

-Legumes

-Cereal grains

-Starchy vegetables

-Processed foods

-Salt

-Dairy

-Processed sugar

-Distilled vegetable oils

As stated above, each version of the diet differs in its limits. Hence, some foods accept low-fat dairy produce and yams as a part of the meal. All adaptations of the regime promote lean proteins, fruit, vegetables and good fats from sources such as nuts (except for peanuts), seeds, and grass-fed meat.

Consequently, the Paleo diet is quite low in carbohydrates but loaded with protein and healthy fats, which help the body add necessary fiber, vitamins, minerals, and phytochemicals. Nothing like other dietary regimens, the Paleo diet does not encourage seasoned cold cut meats yet allows the follower to consume fruits and vegetables that have alkaline in them.

The diet is not low in fat, but in its place, the regime advances the addition of natural fats from grass-fed cattle, fish, and seafood, as well as nuts, seeds, and their oils to the digestive system. The prohibition of such an extensive assortment of foods such as grains, dairy, processed foods, and sugar suggests the diet may lead to significant weight loss.

Chapter 2: Getting Started on your Challenge

There can be no denying it, any time you set out to change a significant part of your routine, it is a challenge. And that is very fitting for the 30-day Paleo Challenge. Hence the name challenge is used in the title. In this chapter, we will examine all of the nuances and idiosyncrasies for you to come out on your Paleo Challenge on top.

Buy the Right Produce

It may seem like a heavy dose of common sense that we are dishing out here, but there is no way that you can begin this challenge on proper footing unless you start off with the adequate product in the first place. There are certain things that you should have on your grocery list and also a few things that you should not. The first things that you should scratch off of that said list are anything containing a heavy dose of sugar, salt, or wheat based sorghum. These are just carb buildings nuisances so you should toss them at your earliest convenience.

You should also throw to the wayside much of your supply of heavily processed grain products. Unfortunately for most of us, this means getting rid of about 90% of our pantry! We are a country that loves our processed foods plain and simple. But to be successful on this diet, you will have to part with them! I can remember back to when I first tried the paleo challenge, and just how many of these over-processed foods I had to ditch just to get started.

From the get-go I had to empty out much of the contents of my cupboards and replace them with foods that were more paleo friendly. Instead of stockpiling heavily processed grains you should load up on some all-natural grass-fed meats such as lamb, chicken, goat, and beef. Animals that are strictly grass fed are free of the chemicals, hormones, and other toxins that make up most of the rest of our heavily processed and overtaxed food supply.

Grass-fed meats also offer many other benefits such as more omega-3 fatty acids that aid in the reduction of heart disease and have even been shown to prevent cancer. It is for this reason that you see so many vitamins on store shelves touting that they are loaded to the max with "omega 4". But you don't have to pop pills to get this benefit folk, all you have to do is eat it! And the recipes in this book make full use of meat that came from these grass-fed animals, significantly bolstering your health in the process.

Along with grass-fed meat from livestock animals, you should also get some cans of salmon, sardines, and tuna. You may have heard fish being referred to as a "brain food" and this is no accident. Fish are a central store of iodine. Iodine helps to regulate our thyroid gland as well as facilitate brain function. Our Paleolithic ancestors were dependent on fish for this very reason. Fish can help control neural capacity and with the endless variety of recipes available for the Paleo challenge, fish and fish products should not be overlooked.

Next, to these meat staples, you should also make sure that you have plenty of fruit packed up in your cupboards as well. But the veggies that you should avoid are those items full of starch such as potatoes, legumes, and lentils. People are surprised by this, but you should also nix any peanut consumption as well.

But interestingly, although you can't eat peanuts, peanut oil is an excellent part of the 30-Day Paleo Challenge. Along with sesame oil, olive oil, coconut oil, and a few others. These cooking oils are highly nutritious and should be on your list. You can find them at most department and health food stores. Buy the right produce folks!

Make a Food Calendar

While we aren't precisely tracking carbs, or counting calories during the 30-Day Paleo Challenge, we need to be mindful of the fact that we should have a general idea of what kinds of meals we are going to eat throughout the week. And this means creating what is called a "Food Calendar" a calendar in which you put your specific meal plans down on each calendar day of the week so that you can see them and know them without any difficulty. This is of great use in the 30-day Paleo Challenge. Just manage your routine, and you can do the rest!

But if it is indeed a meal plan that you need to keep track of, you should move towards sectioning off your refrigerator and categorize precisely what it is that you would like to eat. One of the easiest ways to do this is to demarcate on your calendar days; a time during the day for Breakfast, a time during the day for Lunch, and a time during the day for Dinner. Once you have these headings in place, you can then put them down in real time on the calendar.

If you are a visual person like I am, having this daily reminder will help you out tremendously. And whatever it is that you plan out on your food calendar does not have to be set in stone either; this is just a template to get you started. You should make your list and check it twice, so you can make sure that you remain on task for the 30-day challenge from beginning to end.

Be Careful with Restaurants

Restaurants are the number one diet breaker known to man. And this is most especially the case with the Paleo diet. Since the Paleo diet requires you to eat some particular foods and food combinations, most restaurants will find it difficult to accommodate these demands. It is for this reason—if it is possible—I would recommend swearing off all restaurants until you successfully finish the 30-day paleo challenge.

But if you have no choice in the matter, and absolutely must eat out from time to time, I would recommend sticking to the rawest roughage that you can. This means very strict greens and prime meat. It may take some specific bartering with the restaurant establishment, but it can be done! They might ask you a lot of questions, and you just might find yourself on the spot

I can remember a time I went to a local steakhouse and had to order a specialty made salad because nothing else on the menu made sense. The waitress was friendly enough, but it took two back and forth maneuvers between me, her, and the kitchen chefs to get it right! It took little extra time, but it was worth it since I was able to get through the evening without breaking my 30-day Paleo Challenge.

Chapter 3: Going paleo way

To go Paleo, you need to avoid grains, potatoes, legumes, dairy, refined and processed products, certain vegetable oils, and refined sugar. Instead, focus on fish, grass-fed meats, fruits, and vegetables. Fresh organic produce from a local source is even better. Unlike what you may have heard, the Paleo Diet is not a strict raw-food diet, and food can be eaten either raw or cooked. Practitioners encourage a great deal of variety on the menu to ensure the proper balance of vitamins and minerals.

The health benefits of the diet are many. It will:

Reduce the quantities of stored fat, thereby causing weight loss and toning.

Fill you up with antioxidants, phytonutrients, and other vitamins through a significant amount of fruit you'll be consuming.

Improve brain function, by way of providing essential vitamins and proteins such as omega 3, due to the diet's high quantity of fresh fish. Omega 3 fatty acids are critical for brain development and healthy eyes and heart.

What you won't need to do with this diet is count your calories, or control your portions (Do you think the prehistoric man ever counted their calories?). Instead, this diet relies solely on the foods that you eat to induce these health benefits.

How paleo works

You only take out all of the processed food that early man never ate. Yes, all of it. Dairy, refined sugar, chemicals, processed food. You clean your body of all the additional fuel that is storing itself on your hips and heart as fat. Many modern diseases can be prevented by merely eating healthily, so why complicate your life?

Paleo is all about natural food. You eliminate the overly-processed supermarket meals and gain your energy from healthy eating, the sun and wind, and freedom. Sounds romantic? It is. Let's start with what to avoid so that you can be joyful later.

Chapter 4: Types of Paleo Diets

One of the most significant features of the Paleo diet is that it can be tailored to your exact health requirements or conditions, such as food allergies, religious practices, or moral restraints. It can settle into any nutrient requirements the body needs at each point of your life, and thus it can, in due course, facilitate success.

1. Basic Paleo

The traditional, standard Paleo diet rejects grains, dairy, soy, and refined and processed foods. It also omits bogus fats, in addition to vegetable oils that are excessively processed.

2. 80/20 Paleo

This is most likely what some would regard as the "traditional Paleo."

When Paleo was initially growing to be accepted, some supporters advised being Paleo 80% of the time, while saving the remaining 20% for much-loved non-Paleo foods.

This approach can be adopted by people who are in the Paleo lifestyle if they are a family unit or persons who have already accomplished their physical condition targets.

3. Auto-immune Paleo

The auto-immune etiquette, also branded as Auto-immune Paleo (AIP), is an adaptation of the Paleo diet that is free of particular foods related to inflammatory reactions, particularly for people with persistent and auto-immune conditions, such as fibromyalgia, lupus eczema, multiple sclerosis, rheumatoid arthritis, IBS, and Crohn's disease.

Nightshades, which includes potatoes, tomatoes, eggplants, and peppers, are avoided, alongside seeds, nuts, and eggs.

People who are hypersensitive to these foodstuffs can thrive on the AIP, in addition to everybody who is beginning to adopt Paleo diets when living with illness, poor digestion, or irritation. Some people will continually live on the AIP diet, while others will in due course, evolve to fundamental Paleo.

4. Ketogenic Paleo

Ketogenic Paleo is mainly practiced by those who have an enormous amount of weight to lose, diabetics, or bodybuilders. It can, moreover, be made use of to keep up a wellness arrangement for epilepsy.

6. The Pegan Diet

Pegan is a conjunction of "Paleo Vegan" and is precisely what it sounds like: a Paleo regime that prohibits all animal-sourced products and is entirely vegan. Despite the fact that fundamental Paleo doctrines are founded on the accommodating advantages of animal foodstuffs that have been morally reared and supplied, this adaptation of Paleo centers on plant protein and fats, and is chiefly for those who are ethically or conscientiously against ingesting animals. For this reason, Paleo specialists do not advise a Vegan diet, especially for auto-immune or persistent health difficulties.

If the Paleo regimen is too radical for a newcomer, please initiate by following a simple Paleo diet. This will allow the body and mind some time to adjust to the new limitations, which can be somewhat alarming at first. Giving up and not consuming dairy and grains are huge steps, and are not easy to do. So, as an alternative, do not impose harsh restrictions when you start your Paleo diet. Just try out with an essential Paleo diet.

Chapter 5: Benefits of the Paleo

Diet 1. Weight loss

The Paleo diet is a low-carbohydrate diet deliberately. Merely getting rid of junk and refined food will radically cut carbohydrate ingestion to stimulate weight loss.

By restricting carbohydrates, shedding unnecessary weight is possible. Here is where Paleo plays a significant part in reducing waistlines and stubborn fat by burning excess fat.

2. Brain Enhancement

One of the most beautiful supplies of protein and fat recommended by the Paleo diet emerges from wild salmon.

A Paleo diet which is based on cold water fish can enhance brain function, due to the omega three fatty acids.

3. Improved Gut Health

Sugar, artificial fats, and other refined edibles cause inflammation inside the intestinal tract. Sadly, when an unnecessary amount of processed foods meet with a lot of anxiety, the result may be "leaky gut syndrome;" which means that the intestinal walls are infringed, and things that do not leave the passage end up seeping out. Apparently, a person wants to keep our digestive food in the gastrointestinal tract until it is all set to be brought to your cells so that energy can be produced.

Eating Paleo can help indefinitely with the problem, because processed food and sugars are eliminated, leaving little to no chance of a mishap occurring.

The Paleo regime proposes eating grass-fed meats and considers eggs also very important. This means that birds and cattle can wander freely and peacefully during their whole lives. Cows and chickens will ramble the grazing land as one, as this generates synergy. In the natural world, chickens will trail cows and eat the larvae and bugs living under cow dung. Cowpats will decompose, which fertilizes the grass, which in turn, supplies food for the cow. This diet is perfect for the natural world. Moreover, it provides an enormous amount of nutrients when consumed, due to the animals' healthy eating. It is the circle of life at its best.

5. Catch-All Vitamins and Minerals

The Paleo diet advocates consuming the "rainbow" itself. Vegetables are a significant component of the lifestyle. Eating vegetables and fruits when in the season is the best way to stock up on the essential nutrients. The diverse colors of plants indicate the presence of a variety of nutrients.
By having a rainbow, it is guaranteed that one will get all the vitamins needed.

6. Cut the Threat of Disease

The Paleo diet is not necessarily the best for many people, but people tend to ignore that the main point is to steer clear of foods that can probably affect your well-being.
The Paleo diet makes it easy to avoid bad food: eat what a cave dweller would be able to eat.

In this way, consumption of fresh and whole food can considerably reduce the threat of numerous diseases and the factors that cause them.

7. Better Digestion and Absorption

This particular regime advocate eating food that we adapted to over thousands of years ago. This means that these foods were consumed in their purest form and therefore were easy on digestion.

If digestive problems are recurring, trying an austere Paleo diet for at least a month will make you feel healthier for sure.

8. Fewer Allergies

In this diet, you are advised to restrict food items that are allergens for some people. Some are unable to digest seeds, grains, and dairy, which is the reason why the Paleo diet advocates the elimination of these food products when most menus do not skip these 'trigger' foods, and the people affected are considerably more in control of their allergies when under the Paleo regime.

9. Reduce Inflammation

Studies show that inflammation is the primary issue behind cardiovascular disease. The Paleo diet focuses solely on food items that are anti-inflammatory, thereby reducing the risk of heart disease significantly.

The presence of omega three fatty acids is one of the reasons for which the Paleo diet is anti-inflammatory. Grass-fed animals have a much-improved percentage of omega 3 and 6, along with the intake of recommended fruits and vegetables.

10. New Energy

Energy drinks are widely favorite these days, which leads to the question of why they became such a demand so fast. It is because as a person's diet deteriorates, their energy levels plummet too.

Breakfast cereals and any food that is advertised as giving energy drain you of it. When following the Paleo diet, there has been a reported significant increase in strength due to the high protein content.

11.   Healthy   Cells

Each cell in the body is made with a combination of saturated and unsaturated fat, and the cells count on a proper equilibrium of these fats so that the messages are accurately sent in and out. The Paleo diet offers ideal equality of lipids, since both saturated and unsaturated fats exist in adequate quantities in the Paleo diet, while other foods lack one or the additional fat.

12. Increased Insulin Sensitivity

When a person regularly supplies their body with sugary and junk food, in time the body numbs itself to this food, as it does not indeed desire or require it. This is where the surplus sugar and carbohydrates store up – because the cells do not have a specific use for their energy, the cells reject this sugar. This leads to insulin sensitivity where the body will be inept in identifying when the cells are filled or not.

13. Confines Intake of Fructose

Paleo diets make the human body absorb fructose differently from other carbohydrates. For this reason, you must avoid consuming too many fruit portions when you follow the Paleo diet. Choose fruits best for you.

Unless advised by an expert, limit yourself to 2-3 portions of fruit every day.

Chapter 6: Paleo diet Recipes to get you started

Breakfast recipes

1. Breakfast Tomato and Eggs

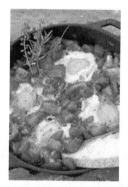

It's going to become one of your favorite paleo meals in no time. It's delicious!

Servings: 2

Preparation time: 15 minutes

Ingredients:
- Two eggs
- Two tomatoes
- Salt and black pepper to the taste
- One teaspoon parsley, finely chopped

Directions:

1. Cut tomatoes tops, scoop flesh and arrange them on a lined baking sheet.

2. Crack an egg into each tomato.

3. Season with salt and pepper.

4. Introduce them in the oven at 350 degrees F and bake for 30 minutes.

5. Take tomatoes out of the oven, divide between plates, season with more salt and pepper, sprinkle parsley at the end and serve.

Enjoy!

2. Breakfast Paleo Muffins

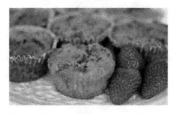

It's a paleo breakfast that will provide you enough energy to face a busy day at work. Just try it!

Servings: 4

Preparation time: 40 minutes

Ingredients:

- 1 cup kale, chopped
- ¼ cup chives, finely chopped

- ½ cup almond milk
- Six eggs
- Salt and black pepper to the taste
- Some coconut oil for greasing the muffin cups

Directions:

1. In a bowl, mix eggs with chives and kale and whisk very well.

2. Add salt and black pepper to the taste and almond milk and stir well.

3. Divide this into eight muffin cups after you've greased it with some coconut oil.

4. Introduce this in a preheated oven at 350 degrees F and bake for 30 minutes.

5. Take muffins out of the oven, leave them to cool down, transfer them to plates and serve warm.

Enjoy!

3. Paleo Banana Pancakes

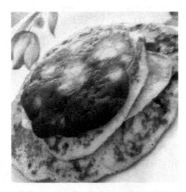

These are so healthy and delicious! You will enjoy making them, and you will love eating them!

Servings: 2

Preparation time: 30 minutes

Ingredients:
- 4 eggs
- A pinch of salt
- Two bananas, peeled and chopped
- ¼ teaspoon baking powder
- Cooking spray

Directions:
1. In a bowl, mix eggs with chopped bananas, a pinch of salt and baking powder and whisk well.
2. Transfer this to your food processor and blend very well.

3.   Heat up a pan over medium-high heat after you've sprayed it with some cooking oil.

4.   Add some of the pancakes batter, spread in the pan, cook for 1 minute, flip and cook for 30 seconds and transfer to a plate.

5. Serve and enjoy!

4. Plantain Pancakes

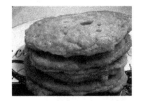

These are not only very tasty! These paleo pancakes also look excellent!

Servings: 1

Preparation time: 20 minutes

Ingredients:
- 3 eggs
- ¼ cup coconut flour
- ¼ cup coconut water
- One teaspoon coconut oil
- ½ plantain, peeled and chopped
- ¼ teaspoon cream of tartar
- ¼ teaspoon baking soda
- A pinch of salt

- ¼ teaspoon chai spice
- One tablespoon shaved coconut, toasted for serving
- One tablespoon coconut milk for serving

Directions:

1. In your food processor, mix eggs with a pinch of salt, coconut water and flour, plantain, cream of tartar, baking soda and chai spice and blend well.

2. Heat up a pan with the coconut oil over medium heat, add ¼ cup pancake batter, spread evenly, cook until it becomes golden, flip pancake and cook for one more minute and transfer to a plate.

3. Serve pancakes with shaved coconut and coconut milk. Enjoy!

5. Paleo Baked Muffins

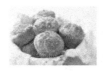

I know that for many dieters anything associated with muffins (or perhaps muffin tops) are readily avoided. But these muffins are specially made for the paleo diet and do not contain any ingredient that you have to worry about. The almond flour that they are made with make them very nutritious, and they also happen to taste great! So go ahead and eat up!

Here are the exact ingredients:
- 1 cup of almond flour
- One teaspoon of baking powder
- ¼ teaspoon of salt
- ¼ cup of butter
- ½ a bowl of water
- Three eggs

1. To get started putting your oven temperature at 345 degrees and grease the cups of a muffin tin with either coconut oil, or some other kind of low-fat cooking spray.
2. Put this muffin tin to the side and get out a mixing bowl. Inside this bowl add your cup of almond flour, your teaspoon of baking powder, ¼ cup of butter, three eggs, ½ cup of water and ¼ teaspoon of salt.
3. Mix these ingredients well. After they've become nicely mixed, dump the mix into the cups of the greased muffin tin you had just set to the side, and place the muffin tin in the oven.
4. Your paleo baked muffins should be thoroughly cooked after only about 10 minutes or so.
5. A couple of these muffins in the morning is a healthy and refreshing way to start your day!

6. Coconut Flour Waffles

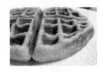

Ok, so the caveman probably didn't have a waffle iron, but that doesn't mean this breakfast item is not paleo diet compatible. This recipe utilizes only strictly paleo ingredients, with the healthy staple of coconut flour as its main component. Just put these bad boys in a waffle iron, and you will have yourself the best Paleolithic inspired waffles you could ever come by!

Here are the main ingredients:
- 1 cup of coconut flour
- Three eggs
- ½ teaspoon of baking soda
- ½ cup of honey
- ½ cup vanilla extract
- ½ teaspoon salt

1. To get started, take out that old waffle iron that you have been hiding, plug it in and get it warmed up.
2. While your equipment gets warmed up go ahead and get out a mixing bowl add your three eggs, ½ teaspoon of baking soda, ½ cup of honey, 2 cups of vanilla extract.

3. Once these ingredients are mixed add your cup of coconut flour, and stir it into the components of the mixing bowl until it is all thoroughly combined.
4. This mixture will constitute your batter.
5. After your batter is established, go to your waffle iron and spray it well with an excellent fat-free, paleo friendly, coconut cooking spray so that your mixture doesn't stick to the waffle iron.
6. Once this preparation has been made you should then get out a medium-sized spoon and begin to scoop up your batter into your waffle iron. Close your iron and let your waffle cook until it is nice and brown.
7. This is a paleo bed and breakfast so good that even the crankiest of cave dwellers will get out of bed for it!

7. The Paleo Omelet

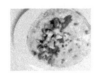

You don't have to eat pterodactyl eggs in order satisfy your paleo cravings because this dish from the Neolithic will make your day! It meets the classic bacon and egg cravings yet the healthy coconut oil this dish is cooked with won't wreck your diet. Many aspects of what makes paleo—well, paleo—is in preparation. And the Paleo Omelet is a shining testament to that fact.

Here are the exact ingredients:
- Two eggs
- Two strips of diced bacon
- ½ pound of diced mushrooms
- ¼ cup of coconut oil

1. Take a medium saucepan and put it over low heat. Now dump your diced bacon with your coconut oil and begin marinating the meat in your pot.
2. After you have done this, add your diced mushrooms and then stir the whole mixture together for a minute or so.
3. Next, add your two eggs and stir the eggs in as well. Continue stirring the mixture until everything is thoroughly blended into one big circle of ingredients. Now let this cook for another minute or so until the eggs solidify and bond with the other components, making for one tasty paleo omelet!

8. Pine Nut Scrambled Eggs

This is a tasty blend of hunter gatherer style pine nuts mixed with mushrooms and scrambled eggs! All food that could have easily been forged by our Paleolithic forefathers! This recipe provides a satisfying blend of nuts, chives, mushrooms, and berries. The taste and texture are fantastic. As soon as you take a bite and hear that pine nut crunch, you know that you are in for a treat!

Here are the exact ingredients:
- Two eggs
- One tablespoon chopped chives
- ½ cup of diced mushrooms
- ½ tablespoon coconut oil
- ½ tablespoon pine nuts

1. As usual with these kinds of recipes, begin the task by coating your frying pan with coconut oil over high heat.
2. While your oil warms up, go ahead and break your eggs open and empty their contents into the container.
3. After you have done this, dump your diced mushrooms, your ½ tablespoon of pine nuts, and your tablespoon of chopped chives.
4. Your Pine Nut Scrambled Eggs are now ready for business!

9. Chicken and Veggie Breakfast

This dish is useful for anyone who likes their chicken and veggies! This is a bit of a departure from the traditional breakfast, but if you feel like you need a break from eggs and bacon, this one is a good one for you! Using only the best lean chicken meat, along with a delectable blend of veggies, this breakfast dish will make you happy you woke up in the morning!

Here are the exact ingredients:
- ¼ cup of olive oil
- ½ cup chopped onion
- ½ cup chopped garlic
- ¼ cup of chopped asparagus
- 1 cup chopped carrots
- ½ cup of shredded chicken
- ¼ cup of fresh, chopped spinach

1. Put a medium pan on a burner set to high heat.
2. Place chopped onions, and chopped garlic into the pan and periodically stir the ingredients as they cook.

3. Now add your chopped asparagus and carrots to the pan and stir them as they prepare for a few more minute as well.
4. Next, add your ½ cup of shredded chicken to the pan and let it cook for a couple of minutes as well.
5. Turn off your burner, and add your fresh, chopped spinach, making it cook from the residual steam that forms.
6. Once you have done this, place a cover on the pan and drip your lemon juice onto the ingredients. This chicken and veggie breakfast are ready to enjoy.

10. Early Morning Salmon

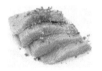

This one isn't on your typical breakfast menu, but it is a Paleolithic treat all the same! Tasty fresh fish coupled with delicious mushrooms, tomatoes, and a classy blend of herbs and spices, this recipe is not to be missed! Try it out at least once during your 30 Day Paleo Challenge!

Here are the exact ingredients:
- 3 Salmon Fillet
- ¼ cup of olive oil
- ¼ cup chopped fresh dill

- ¼ cup of paprika
- ¼ cup of ground black pepper
- ½ cup of white mushrooms
- 1 cup of diced tomatoes

1. In a medium saucepan, place a steamer basket and add 1 inch of water to the pan.
2. Let this come to a boil, reduce your heat to just a simmer and then put your fish in the steamer and let it cook for about 20 minutes or until the fish starts to brown.
3. After you have done this, take out a separate pan and put in your olive oil.
4. Next, add your ¼ cup of chopped fresh dill, your ¼ cup of paprika, and your ½ cup of mushrooms.
5. Stir fry this mixture for a few minutes before adding in your tomatoes.
6. Stir for another few minutes and then remove the pan from the heat altogether, and turn your burner off.
7. As soon as your fish are done the cooking, remove them as well and add your mushroom and tomato mix on top of your fish.
8. Get up early for this morning salmon treat!

11. Paleo Power Breakfast

If you are primarily active throughout the day, this high protein breakfast will give you the energy you need for your busy morning routine! Cooked in abundant olive oil, freshly chopped turkey is roasted and marinated in tomatoes, onions, and basil! Just add a couple of eggs, and you've got yourself a real Paleolithic power broker! Give this recipe a chance and you won't regret it!

Here are the exact ingredients:
- ¼ cup of olive oil
- 1 cup of chopped turkey breast (already cooked)
- ½ cup diced tomato
- ½ cup diced onions
- ¼ cup dried basil
- Two eggs

1. Put your frying pan on a burner set to medium heat. Now take out a small plastic bowl, add your eggs, and whisk them into oblivion!
2. Stir these eggs as well as you can until they consist of one fine egg paste. Now pour these eggs into your pan and let them cook on medium heat for about 1 and a half minute, as you periodically lift up the edges with a plastic utensil (spoon or spatula) just to make sure that the egg mixture doesn't stick to the pan.
3. Next, add your onions, tomatoes, and turkey breast.
4. Fold your egg over these ingredients so that the cooked egg covers them like a crepe (or taco).

5. Let the entire entrée cook like this for about three more minutes. Now all you have to do is cut the combination in half and put the pieces onto a large plate.
6. All of these recipes are great for breakfast or any other time!

12. Paleo Sweet Potato Waffles

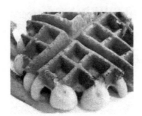

You only need a few ingredients, and you have to follow some simple directions, and you will enjoy some delicious paleo waffles in no time!

Servings: 4

Preparation time: 30 minutes

Ingredients:
- Two sweet potatoes, peeled and finely grated
- Two tablespoons melted coconut oil
- Three eggs
- One teaspoon cinnamon powder
- ½ teaspoon nutmeg, ground
- Some applesauce for serving

Directions:

1. In a bowl, mix eggs with sweet potatoes, coconut oil, cinnamon and nutmeg and whisk very well.

2. Cook waffles in your waffle iron, arrange them on plates and serve with applesauce drizzled on top.

Enjoy!

Lunch recipes

13. Paleo Beef Soup

Your family will enjoy eating this flavored soup! You will love it too!

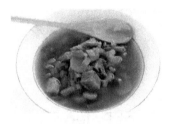

Servings: 6

Preparation time: 10 minutes Cooking time: 1 hour

Ingredients:

- 1 pound beef, ground
- 1 pound sausage, sliced
- 4 cups beef stock
- 30 ounces canned tomatoes, diced
- One green bell pepper, chopped
- Three zucchinis, chopped

- 1 cup celery, chopped
- One teaspoon Italian seasoning
- ½ yellow onion, chopped
- ½ teaspoon oregano, dried
- ½ teaspoon basil, dried
- ¼ teaspoon garlic powder
- Salt and black pepper to the taste

Directions:

1.   cook until it browns and drains excess fat.

2.   Add tomatoes, zucchini, bell pepper, celery, onion, Italian seasoning, basil, oregano, garlic powder, salt, pepper to the taste and the stock, stir, bring to a boil, reduce heat to medium-low and simmer for 1 hour.

3.   Enjoy!

14. Root Paleo Soup

The root veggies you'll use for this soup taste fantastic! The soup is perfect!

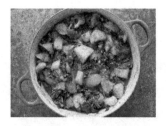

Servings: 8

Preparation time: 10 minutes Cooking time: 1 hour and 30 minutes

Ingredients:
- One sweet onion, chopped
- Two tablespoons butter
- Five carrots, chopped
- Three parsnips, chopped
- Three beets, chopped
- Three bacon slices
- 1-quart chicken stock
- Salt and black pepper to the taste
- 2 quarts water
- ½ teaspoon chili flakes
- One tablespoon mixed thyme and rosemary

Directions:
1.   Heat up a Dutch oven with the butter over medium-high heat, add onion, stir and cook for 5 minutes.
2.   Add carrots, parsnips, beets, bacon, chicken stock and water and stir.
3.   Also add salt, pepper to the taste, chili flakes, thyme, and rosemary, stir again, bring to a boil, reduce heat to medium-low and simmer for 1 hour and 30 minutes.
4.   Pour into soup bowls and serve hot.
Enjoy!

15. Delightful Chicken Soup

This fantastic paleo chicken soup is such an elegant option for a fancy lunch!

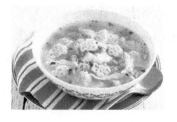

Servings: 6

Preparation time: 15 minutes Cooking time: 30 minutes

Ingredients:

- Two celery stalks, chopped
- ½ cup coconut oil
- Two carrots, chopped
- ½ cup arrowroot
- 6 cups chicken stock
- One teaspoon dry parsley
- ½ cup water
- One bay leaf
- Salt and black pepper to the taste
- ½ teaspoon dry thyme
- 1 and ½ cups coconut milk
- 3 cups chicken meat, already cooked and cubed

Directions:

1. Heat up a soup pot with the oil over medium-high heat, add carrots and celery, stir and cook for 10 minutes.
2. Add stock, stir and bring to a boil.

3.   In a bowl, mix arrowroot with ½ cup water and whisk well.

4.   Add this to soup and also add parsley, salt, pepper to the taste, bay leaf and thyme.

5.   Stir and cook everything for 15 minutes.

6.   Add chicken meat and coconut milk, stir, cook one more minute, take off heat, pour into soup bowls and serve.

Enjoy!

16. Paleo Lemon and Garlic Soup

It is an exotic style soup! It's also straightforward to make!

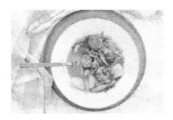

Serving: 4

Preparation time: 10 minutes Cooking time: 20 minutes

Ingredients:

- 6 cups shellfish stock
- One tablespoons garlic, finely minced
- One tablespoon ghee
- Two eggs
- ½ cup lemon juice
- Salt and white pepper to the taste

- One tablespoon arrowroot powder
- Cilantro, finely chopped for serving

Directions:

1.   Heat up a pot with the ghee over medium-high heat, add garlic, stir and cook for 2 minutes.

2.   Add stock but reserve ½ cup, stir and bring to a simmer.

3.   Meanwhile, in a bowl, mix eggs with salt, pepper, reserved stock, lemon juice and arrowroot and whisk very well.

4.   Pour this into soup, stir and cook for a few minutes.

5.   Ladle into bowls and serve with chopped cilantro on top. Enjoy!

17. Rich Paleo Soup

It's a very creamy soup with such an intense color! Taste it today!

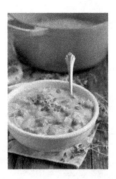

Servings: 3

Preparation time: 10 minutes Cooking time: 0

Ingredients:

- One avocado, pitted and chopped
- One cucumber, cut
- Two bunches spinach
- One and ½ cups watermelon, chopped
- One bunch cilantro, roughly chopped
- Juice of 2 lemons
- ½ cup coconut amino
- ½ cup lime juice

Directions:

1. In your kitchen blender, mix cucumber with avocado and pulse well.
2. Add cilantro, spinach, and watermelon and blend again well.
3. Add lemon and lime juice and coconut amino and pulse a few more times.
4. Transfer to soup bowls and enjoy!

18. Paleo Lamb and Coconut Stew

It's an Indian style stew you should make for you and your loved ones as soon as possible!

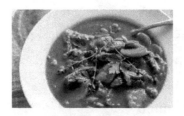

Servings: 4

Preparation time: 15 minutes Cooking time: 1 hour and 50 minutes

Ingredients:
- 1 and ½ pounds lamb meat, diced
- One tablespoon coconut oil
- ½ red chili, seedless and chopped
- One brown onion, chopped
- Three garlic cloves, minced
- Two celery sticks, chopped
- 2 and ½ teaspoons garam masala powder
- One teaspoon fennel seeds
- Salt and black pepper to the taste
- 1 and ¼ teaspoons turmeric
- 1 and ½ teaspoons ghee
- 14 ounces canned coconut milk
- 1 and ½ tablespoons coconut milk
- 1 cup water
- One tablespoon lemon juice

- Two carrots, chopped
- A handful parsley leaves, finely chopped

Directions:

1. Heat up a pan with the oil over medium-high heat, add lamb, stir and brown for 4 minutes.
2. Add celery, chili and onion, stir and cook 1 minute.
3. Reduce heat to medium, add garam masala, garlic, ghee, fennel, and turmeric, stir and cook 1 minute.
4. Add salt, pepper to the taste, tomato paste, coconut milk, and water, stir, bring to a boil, reduce heat to low, cover and cook for 1 hour.
5. Add carrots and cook for 40 minutes more, stirring from time to time.
6. Add lemon juice and parsley, stir, take off heat, transfer to bowls and serve.
7. Enjoy!

19. Paleo Veggie Stew

It's a delicious spring dish that proves you don't need meat every day!

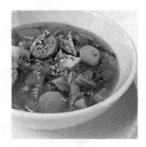

Serving: 4

Preparation time: 10 minutes Cooking time: 20 minutes

Ingredients:

- 4 pounds mixed root vegetables (parsnips, carrots, rutabagas, potatoes, beets, celery root, turnips), chopped
- Six tablespoons extra virgin olive oil
- One garlic head, cloves separated and peeled
- ½ cup yellow onion, chopped
- Salt and black pepper to the taste
- 28 ounces canned tomatoes, peeled and cut
- One tablespoon tomato paste
- 2 cups kale leaves, torn
- One teaspoon oregano, dried
- Tabasco sauce for serving

Directions:

1. In a baking dish, mix all root vegetables with salt, pepper, half of the oil and garlic, toss to coat, introduce in the oven at 450 degrees G and roast them for 45 minutes.
2. Heat up a pot with the rest of the oil over medium-high heat, add onions and cook for 2-3 minutes stirring often.
3. Add tomato paste, stir and cook one more minute.
4. Add tomatoes and their liquid, some salt and pepper and the oregano, stir, bring to a simmer, reduce heat to low and cook until veggies become roasted.
5. Take root vegetables out of the oven, add them to the pot and stir.
6. Add kale, stir and cook for 5 minutes.
7. Add Tabasco sauce to the taste, mix, transfer to bowls and serve.
8. Enjoy!

20. Paleo French Chicken Stew

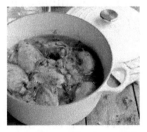

This chicken stew smells unbelievable, and it tastes even better!

Serving: 4

Preparation time: 10 minutes Cooking time: 20 minutes

Ingredients:

- Ten garlic cloves, peeled
- 30 black olives, pitted
- 2 pounds chicken pieces
- 2 cups chicken stock
- 28 ounces canned tomatoes, chopped
- Two tablespoon rosemary, chopped
- Two tablespoons parsley leaves, chopped
- Two tablespoons basil leaves, chopped
- Salt and black pepper to the taste
- A drizzle of extra virgin olive oil

Directions:
1. Heat up a pot with some olive oil over medium-high heat, add chicken pieces, salt, and pepper to the taste and cook for 4 minutes, stirring often.
2. Add garlic, stir and brown for 2 minutes.
3. Add chicken stock, tomatoes, olives, thyme, and rosemary, stir, cover pot and bake in the oven at 325 degrees F for 1 hour.
4. Add parsley and basil, mix, introduce in the oven again and bake for 45 more minutes.
5. Leave stew to cool down for a few minutes, transfer to plates and serve.
6. Enjoy!

21. Paleo Oxtail Stew

You've never tried something similar! It's insanely good!

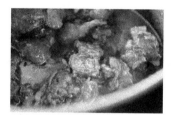

Servings: 8

Preparation time: 15 minutes Cooking time: 6 hours

Ingredients:

- 4 and ½ pounds oxtail, cut into medium chunks
- A drizzle of extra virgin olive oil
- One tablespoon extra virgin olive oil
- Two leeks, chopped
- Four carrots, chopped
- Two celery sticks, chopped
- Four thyme springs, chopped
- Four rosemary springs, chopped
- Four cloves
- Four bay leaves
- Salt and black pepper to the taste
- Two tablespoons flour
- 28 ounces can plum tomatoes, chopped
- 9 ounces red wine
- 1-quart beef stock
- Worcestershire sauce to the taste

Directions:

1. In a roasting pan, mix oxtail with salt and pepper and a drizzle of oil.
2. Toss to coat, introduce the oven at 425 degrees F and bake for 20 minutes.
3. Heat up a pot with one tablespoon oil over medium heat, add leeks, celery, and carrots, stir and cook for 4 minutes.
4. Add thyme, rosemary and bay leaves, stir and cook everything for 20 minutes.
5. Take oxtail out of the oven and leave aside for a few moments.
6. Add flour and cloves to veggies and stir.
7. Also add tomatoes, wine, oxtail and its juices and stock, stir, increase heat to high and bring to a boil.
8. Introduce pot in the oven at 325 degrees F and bake for 5 hours.
9. Take stew out of the oven, leave aside for 10 minutes, take oxtail out of the pot and discard bones.
10. Return meat to pot, add more salt and pepper to the taste and some Worcestershire sauce, stir, transfer to plates and serve.
11. Enjoy!

22. Paleo Eggplant Stew

It's time to teach you how to make the best paleo eggplant stew! Pay attention!

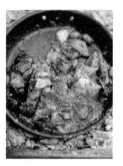

Servings: 3

Preparation time: 10 minutes Cooking time: 30 minutes

Ingredients:

- One eggplant, chopped
- One yellow onion, chopped
- Two tomatoes, chopped
- One teaspoon cumin powder
- Salt and black pepper to the taste
- 1 cup tomato paste
- A pinch of cayenne pepper
- ½ cup water

Directions:

1. Heat up a pan over medium-high heat, add water, tomato paste, salt and pepper, cayenne and cumin and stir well.
2. Add the eggplant, tomato, and onion, stir, bring to a boil, reduce heat to medium and cook for 30 minutes.

3. Take stew off heat, add more salt and pepper if needed, transfer to plates and serve.
4. Enjoy!

23. Paleo Beef Tenderloin with Special Sauce

We don't want to spoil the surprise! We'll allow you to discover step by step how to make this amazing paleo dish!

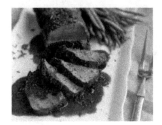

Servings: 4

Preparation time: 10 minutes Cooking time: 40 minutes

Ingredients:
- Three tablespoons Dijon mustard
- 3 pounds beef tenderloin
- Salt and black pepper to the taste
- One tablespoon coconut oil
- Three tablespoons balsamic vinegar
- For the sauce:
- Three tablespoons basil leaves, chopped
- ½ cup parsley leaves, chopped
- Zest of 1 lemon

- Two garlic cloves, finely chopped
- Salt and black pepper to the taste
- ¼ cup extra virgin olive oil

Directions:
1. In a bowl, mix mustard with vinegar, stir very well and leave aside.
2. Season beef with salt and pepper to the taste put in a pan heated with the coconut oil over medium-high heat and cook for 2 minutes on each side.
3. Transfer beef to a baking pan, cover with mustard sauce, introduce in the oven at 475 degrees F and bake for 25 minutes.
4. Meanwhile, in a bowl, mix parsley with basil, lemon zest, garlic, olive oil, salt, and pepper to the taste and whisk very well.
5. Take beef tenderloin out if the oven, leave aside for a few minutes to cool down, slice and divide between plates.
6. Serve with herbs sauce on the side.
7. Enjoy!

24. Paleo Beef Stir Fry

It's an Asian style dish! It's tasty; it's light and straightforward to make at home!

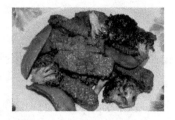

Servings: 4

Preparation time: 10 minutes Cooking time: 20 minutes

Ingredients:
- 10 ounces mushrooms, sliced
- 10 ounces asparagus, sliced
- 1 and ½ pounds beef steak, thinly sliced
- Two tablespoons honey
- 1/3 cup coconut amino
- Two teaspoons apple cider vinegar
- ½ teaspoon ginger, minced
- Six garlic cloves, minced
- One chili, sliced
- One tablespoon coconut oil
- Salt and black pepper to the taste

Directions:

1. In a bowl, mix garlic with coconut amino, honey, ginger, and vinegar and whisk well.
2. Put some water in a pan, heat up over medium-high heat, add asparagus, cook for 3 minutes, transfer to a bowl filled with ice water, drain and leave aside.
3. Heat up a pan with the oil over medium-high heat, add mushrooms, cook for 2 minutes on each side, transfer to a bowl and also leave aside.
4. Heat up the same pan over high heat, add meat, brown for a few minutes and mix with hot pepper.
5. Cook for two more minutes and mix with asparagus, mushrooms and vinegar sauce you've made at the beginning.
6. Stir well, cook for 3 minutes, take off heat, divide between plates and serve.
7. Enjoy!

25. Paleo Pork Dish With Delicious Blueberry Sauce

It's such a juicy and delicious dish! You will love it once you try it!

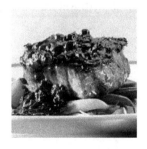

Servings: 4

Preparation time: 10 minutes Cooking time: 30 minutes

Ingredients:

- 1 cup blueberries
- ½ teaspoon thyme, dried
- 2 pounds pork loin
- One tablespoon balsamic vinegar
- ½ teaspoon red chili flakes
- One teaspoon ginger powder
- Salt and black pepper to the taste
- Two tablespoon water

Directions:

1. Put pork loin in a baking dish and season with salt and pepper to the taste.
2. Heat up a pan over medium heat, add blueberries and mix with vinegar, water, thyme, chili flakes and ginger.
3. Stir well, cook for 5 minutes and pour over pork loin.
4. Introduce in the oven at 375 degrees F and bake for 25 minutes.
5. Take pork out of the oven, leave aside for 5 minutes, slice, divide between plates and serve with blueberries sauce.
6. Enjoy!

26. Tasty Paleo Pulled Pork

Are you in the mood for a Mexican dish? Then you should try this one as soon as possible!

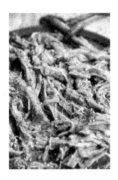

Servings: 4

Preparation time: 12 hours and 10 minutes Cooking time: 8 hours and 20 minutes

Ingredients:
- ½ cup salsa
- ½ cup beef stock
- ½ cup enchilada sauce
- 3 pounds pork shoulder
- Two green chilies, chopped
- One tablespoon garlic powder
- One tablespoon chili powder
- One teaspoon onion powder
- One teaspoon cumin
- One teaspoon paprika
- Salt and black pepper to the taste

Directions:

1. In a bowl, mix chili powder with onion and garlic one.
2. Add cumin, paprika, salt, and pepper to the taste and stir everything.
3. Add pork, rub well and keep in the fridge for 12 hours.
4. Transfer pork to your slow cooker, add enchilada sauce, stock, salsa and green chilies, stir, cover and cook on Low for 8 hours.
5. Transfer pork to a plate, leave aside to cool down and shred.
6. Strain sauce from slow cooker into a pan, bring to a boil over medium heat and simmer for 8 minutes stirring all the time.
7. Add shredded pork to the sauce, stir, reduce heat to medium and cook for 20 more minutes.
8. Divide between plates and serve hot.
9. Enjoy!

27. Paleo Barbeque Ribs

Take a look at this recipe, get all the ingredients and make it for your loved ones tonight!

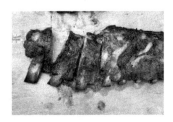

Servings: 4

Preparation time: 15 minutes Cooking time: 2 hours and 47 minutes

Ingredients:

- One tablespoon smoked paprika
- ½ tablespoon onion powder
- ½ tablespoon garlic powder
- ½ teaspoon cayenne pepper
- 4 pounds baby ribs
- 1 cup BBQ sauce
- Two tablespoons raw honey
- Four teaspoons Sriracha
- ¼ cup cilantro, chopped
- ¼ cup chives, chopped
- ¼ cup parsley, chopped
- Salt and black pepper to the taste

Directions:

1. In a bowl, mix paprika with onion powder, garlic powder, salt, pepper and cayenne and stir well.
2. Add ribs, toss to coat and arrange them on a lined baking sheet.
3. Introduce in the oven at 325 degrees F and bake them for 2 hours and 30 minutes.
4. In a bowl, mix BBQ sauce with honey and Sriracha and stir well.
5. Take ribs out of the oven, mix them with BBQ sauce, place them on preheated grill over medium-high heat and cook for 7 minutes on each side.
6. Divide ribs on plates, sprinkle chives, cilantro, and parsley on top and serve.
7. Enjoy!

28. Healthy Taco Salad in A Mason jar

(Prepping time: 10 minutes\ Cooking time: 20 minutes |For two servings)

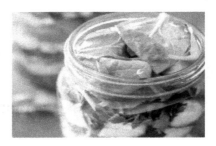

Mason Jars are a delight to have around, especially during the summer season. While usually, we use mason jars to store pickles, in this recipe we are going to be using our Mason Jar to save a finely prepared Taco Salad!

Ingredients:
- One tablespoon of divided up olive oil
- 8 ounce of chicken breast cut into bite-sized portions
- 2 cups of large carrots sliced up
- 1 sliced up sizeable red bell pepper
- ½ a cup of roughly chopped up onion
- Two teaspoon of minced garlic
- Two teaspoon of cumin seed
- One large sized avocado
- One juiced up lime
- 1 cup of salsa
- 2 cup chopped up Roma tomatoes
- ½ a cup of chopped up cucumber

- ½ a cup of roughly chopped up cilantro
- Fresh spinach
- 2 quart of full mouth sized mason jars
- Salt as needed

Preparation: 1) This recipe will first require you to take a large skillet and pour in about ½ tablespoon of olive oil and heat it over medium

2) Toss in the chicken breast and cook them until they are nicely golden brown in texture

3) Pour in a ½ tablespoon of olive oil again into another pan and heat it over medium-high. In this pan, cook the carrots for 3 minute,

4) Bring down the heat to medium and add the pepper, garlic, onion and fry them again until finely charred

5) While the vegetables are begin prepared, take your cumin seed and place it in a small sized dry pan and place it over medium /high heat only to toast them for 2 minutes until golden brown texture

6) Gently transfer them from there to a cutting board just to crush them nicely

7) Take the ground seeds and toss them into the vegetable mix and season using a bit of salt and mix everything before removing the heat

8) Scoop up your avocado and a measure lime juice into the food processor and blend everything until nicely smooth

9) Then, take your mason jar and pour ½ cup of salsa in the bottom.

10) Take your avocado and lime mix and place it on top

11) Then toss the cumin, prepared vegetables, and the chicken

12) Tightly pack everything and follow them with the chopped up tomatoes, cucumbers and top it off with just a bit more cilantro leave

13) Close it up and refrigerate before swallowing up!

29. Crunchy Lettuce Tacos with Chipotle Chicken

(Prepping time: 20 minutes\ Cooking time: 30 minutes |For four servings)

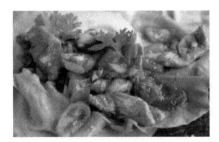

If you are in the mode for chicken but at the same time want something a bit crunchier, don't look further and just go for this one! The Chipotle chicken is finely prepared to go perfectly with your lettuce Tacos.

Ingredients:
- 400g of skinless chicken breast cut into strips
- A splash of olive oil
- One piece of finely sliced red onion
- One piece of 400g tomato tin
- One teaspoon of finely chopped up chipotle
- ½ a teaspoon of cumin
- Pinch of brown sugar
- Lettuce as needed
- Fresh coriander leaves
- Sliced up pickle jalapeno chilies
- Slices of guacamole
- Fresh pieces of tomato slices
- Lime wedges

Preparation:

1) For this recipe, start off by heating up your olive oil in a non-stick frying pan and tossing in the chicken only to fry them until a beautiful golden brown texture has been achieved

2) Keep it aside then and throw in your tomatoes, sugar, cumin, chipotle in another pan and simmer them for about 25 minutes until a beautiful tomato sauce start to get thick edges

3) Into the sauce mixture, toss in your fried chicken and cook for 5 minutes

4) Assemble everything into separate plates and keep them ready for the taco making process

5) Take your taco shell and insert the ingredients according to your desire and squeeze a bit of lemon to top it off.

30. Spicy Cuban Picadillo Lettuce Wraps
(Prepping time: 10 minutes\ Cooking time: 25 minutes |For six servings)

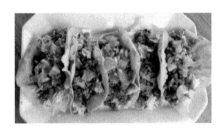

Another recipe involving Lettuce Wraps, but this time a little bit more over the top with finely crafted Paleo suitable Lettuce Tacos!

Ingredients:

For the Picadillo
- 1 pound of grass fed ground beef
- Two tablespoon of coconut oil
- 1.5 cup of diced up onion

- ½ a teaspoon of salt
- One teaspoon of freshly ground black pepper
- One teaspoon of ground cumin
- ½ a teaspoon of ground cinnamon
- One piece of 14 ounces can of whole tomatoes
- ¼ cup of currants
- 2 tablespoon of green olive
- Two tablespoon of drained capers
- 2 tablespoon of olive brine

For the Pico De Gallo

- ½ a cup of minced red onion
- 2/3 cup of diced tomatoes
- Two tablespoon of minced cilantro
- Two teaspoon of fresh lime juice
- Salt as needed

Serving

- Lettuce as required
- Cooked up brown rice
- Chopped up cilantro

Preparation:

1) Take a large sized skillet and place it over medium heat only to toss in the beef and keep stirring it occasionally

2) Pour in the oil to the pan and throw further onions to cook everything until it has been finely softened which should take no more than 3-4 minutes

3) Add the bell pepper and cook for another 3 minutes until nicely fragrant

4) Take another pan and toss in the cooked beef, currants, canned tomatoes, diced olives, olive brine and capers and bring the whole mix to a gentle boil

5) Once boiled, reduce the heat and simmer it for about 10-20 minutes at low temperature

6) On the side, prepare your Pico de Gallo by combining the minced up shallot, cilantro, chopped tomato and lime juice with just a pinch of salt as ending

7) Serve by taking the lettuce leaf and filling it with beef and just a spoonful of rice alongside Pico de Gallo!

31. Healthy California Turkey and Bacon Lettuce Wraps with Basil Mayo
(Prepping time: 10 minutes\ Cooking time: nil |For two servings)

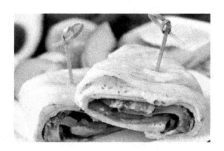

And this recipe, we are mixing up an excellent lettuce wrap with the juicy goodness of Bacon and Basil Mayo for an added Oomph factor.

Ingredients: For the Pico De Gallo

- One head of iceberg lettuce
- Four slices of gluten free deli turkey
- Three slices of gluten-free cooked bacon
- One thinly sliced avocado
- One thinly sliced Roma tomato

Serving

- ½ a cup of gluten free mayonnaise
- Six large pieces of torn basil leaves
- One teaspoon lemon juice
- One chopped up garlic cloves
- Salt as needed
- Pepper as needed

Preparation:

1) Take a small sized food processor to combine all of the ingredients listed under Basil Mayo and process them until very smooth

2) Take your significant lettuce leaves and layer about one slice of turkey and slather alongside the previously prepared Basil Mayo

3) On another layer, add in the second slice of turkey and follow it thoroughly with bacon adding a few slices of tomato and avocado

4) Season them with some pepper and salt and fold them nicely into a burrito 5) Slice in half and serve chilled

32. Savory Steak with Sriracha Lettuce Wraps
(Prepping time: 10 minutes\ Cooking time: 10 minutes |For one servings)

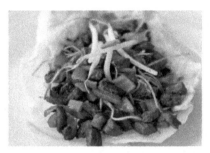

A proper meal cannot be complete without having a few pieces of juicy steak with it, right? This recipe gives you that, and more in the form of Steaks wrapped around in fresh Sriracha Wraps.

Ingredients:
- 1 pound of fajita strips diced up into ½ inch bites
- Large sized onion diced up
- 3 diced up cloves of garlic
- 1 diced up bell pepper
- Two tablespoon of sriracha
- Two teaspoon of coconut
- Sesame oil for drizzle
- Green onions for garnish
- A handful of pea shoots
- Large pieces of romaine leaves

Preparation:

1) Take a hot pan and pour in some oil and heat it for 30 seconds

2) Take your fajita meat and cook them on high for about 2 minutes

3) Add the pepper and onion and keep cooking them on top making sure to toss them occasionally for about 5 minutes until a brown texture has been achieved

4) Then throw in the sesame oil, garlic, sriracha, peas shoot and coconut aminos

5) Once the meat has finally absorbed the sauce, turn off the heat

6) Spoon the mixture up into lettuce cups and top it off with some diced green onions to server hot and savor

33. The Best Cajun Shrimp Noodle Bowl

(Prepping time: 5 minutes\ Cooking time: 15 minutes |For two servings)

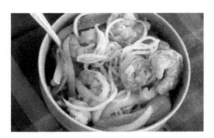

Coming straight from the Mexican tables, this Shrimp Cajun might be a bit spicy, but it's worth every effort! Easily made to satisfy your shrimp lust!

Ingredients: For the Dish

- Three cloves of crushed garlic
- Three tablespoon of grass fed butter
- 20-20 pieces of jumbo shrimps

For the Cajun Seasoning

- One teaspoon of paprika
- Dash of cayenne pepper
- ½ a teaspoon of Himalayan Sea Salt
- Dash of red pepper flakes
- One teaspoon of garlic granules
- One teaspoon of onion powder

For Others

- Two large pieces of spiraled zucchinis
- One sliced red pepper

- One sliced up onion
- One tablespoon of grass fed butter

Preparation:

1) Start off Spiralizing your Zucchini using a fine Spiralizer

2) Take a bowl and toss in the ingredients of the Cajun seasoning and toss the shrimp as well

3) Take a pan and heat up the garlic and butter

4) Toss in the onion and red pepper in that mixture and sauté for about 4 minutes 5) Toss in the Cajun shrimp and cook until nicely opaque

6) Take a separate heating pan heat up the leftover tablespoon of butter and again lightly sauté your Zucchini noodles for about 3 minutes

7) Finely place your Zucchini noodles in a bowl and top it off with your garlic Cajun shrimp and vegetable mixture

8) Add some salt and eat!

34. Quick Paleo Egg Roll In A Bowl

(Prepping time: 10 minutes\ Cooking time: 10 minutes |For two servings)

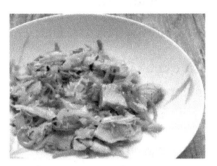

Looking for a quick fix to your Paleo Hunger? Batch up a plate of Paleo egg roll for a rapid lunch to maintain your Paleo diet and also get back to your busy life.

Ingredients:
- One small sized head of a cabbage chopped up into slices
- Two large sized carrots
- One tablespoon of unflavored coconut oil
- 1/3 cup of coconut aminos
- One tablespoon of sesame oil
- Two minced up garlic cloves
- Four pieces of diced up green onions

Preparation:

1) Melt up your coconut oil in a pan over medium-high heat range

2) Toss in the cabbage, followed by the carrots

3) Sautee them until finely softened

4) Toss in the amino and sesame oil afterward

5) Sautee them even more until even further tender, and the sauce has been absorbed 6) Toss in the garlic and keep cooking until translucent and fragrant

7) On top them, toss the green onion

8) Finally, on the side cook your chicken in olive oil/ coconut oil and shred it only to throw in with your salad and eat

35. Simplistic Anti Pasta Salad
(Prepping time: 5 minutes\ Cooking time: nil |For four servings)

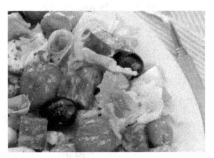

Craving for pasta but can't go for it? Don't frown and go for an Anti-Pasta Salad! This Salad is specifically designed to meet up with your Pasta lust!

Ingredients:
- One large sized head of chopped up romaine
- 4 ounce of strip cut prosciutto
- 4 ounce of cubed up salami

- ½ a cup of artichoke
- ½ a cup of olives
- ½ a cup of hot or sweet peppers
- Italian dressing as required

Preparation:

1) This is a straightforward recipe which only requires you to mix up everything that has been listed throughout and toss them up the Italian dressing

2) Eat up!

Dinner recipes

36. Soft Skillet Chicken Thigh With Butternut Squash

(Prepping time: 15 minutes\ Cooking time: 30 minutes |For 4-6 servings)

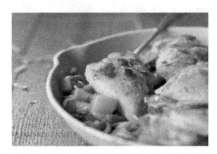

Butternut is pretty famous for their subtle flavor if you have a skillet lying around then plop up some chicken pieces during the dinner sessions to have a happy family meal.

Ingredients:
- ½ a pound of Nitrate free bacon
- Six boneless and skinless chicken thigh
- 2-3 cup of butternut squash cubed up
- Extra Virgin olive oil/ Coconut for frying
- Freshly chopped up sage
- Salt as needed
- Pepper as needed

Preparation:

1) The first step here is to preheat your oven to about 425 degrees Fahrenheit

2) Take a large sized skillet and over medium-high heat, fry up your bacon until it is crispy

3) Take your bacon and place it on the side and crumble it when cooled

4) In the very same skillet, sauté your cubed up butternut squash in bacon grease until tender

5) Season it with pepper and salt

6) Once the squash is softened , remove it from your skillet and place it on a beautiful plate 7) Add your coconut oil to the skillet and if the level of bacon grease is low

8) Toss in the chicken thigh and cook for 10 minutes

9) Season with pepper and salt

10) Flip them over and add your squash

11) Remove the skillet from your stove and place it in your preheated oven

12) Bake for about 12-15 minutes

13) Remove and top with crumbled bacon and sage before serving hot

37. Sweet Paleo Turkey Potato Casserole With Eggplant and Tomato

(Prepping time: 15 minutes\ Cooking time: 60 minutes |For six servings)

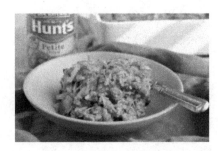

People don't usually consider Eggplant to be a delicious ingredient. But mix it up with sweet potato and turkey, and you got yourself one hell of a meal that has the tanginess of tomato and mixed flavor of eggplant and turkey.

Ingredients: For the Casserole

- 1 pound of extra lean ground turkey
- One medium-sized sweet potato, peeled up and spiralized
- One medium-sized eggplant sliced into ½ inch pieces
- One /4 cup chopped up onion
- One tablespoon of minced up garlic
- One portion of 15 ounces can of petite diced tomatoes
- One can of 8-ounce tomato paste
- ½ a teaspoon of salt
- ½ teaspoon of pepper
- ¼ teaspoon of chili powder

112

- ¼ teaspoon of cumin
- 1/8 teaspoon of oregano
- 1/8 teaspoon of ground cardamom
- ½ a teaspoon of tarragon flakes

For the Sauce

- 1 and a ½ tablespoon of extra virgin olive oil
- 1 cup of unsweet almond milk
- One tablespoon of almond flour
- One tablespoon of coconut flour

Preparation:

1) Preheat your oven to a temperature of 35 0degree Fahrenheit

2) Take an 8x8 inch square casserole dish and spray it with non-stick cooking spray

3) Heat up your large pan over medium level heat and toss in the turkey, onion, and garlic and cook them until finely browed making sure to break apart the turkey with a spatula

4) Stir in your tomato paste and tomatoes to the turkey mixture and add in the sweet potatoes and cook until tender

5) Take your chopped up eggplant in a bowl and toss everything with the seasonings to congregate

6) Finally place the processed eggplant on the bottom part of your casserole dish and top follow it with turkey and sweet potato mix

7) Place it in the oven and let it bake for about 15 minutes

8) While it is being cooked, heat up a small pot and bring it to boil and toss the almond, alongside olive oil and coconut flour

9) Stir in for about 1 minutes until mixture thickens and reduce your heat to medium-high

10) Slowly add the almond milk to the pan while whisking as you stir the mixture

11) Continue whisking for the next 10 minutes until the sauce is reduced to half of its former self

12) Place your casserole back in the oven and cook for about 45 minutes until the top is browned in texture

13) Gently remove everything from the oven and top it up with even more tarragon 14) Slice the mixture into 6 pieces and serve hot

38. Superbly Delicious Paleo Pizza Soup

(Prepping time: 5 minutes\ Cooking time: 30 minutes |For six servings)

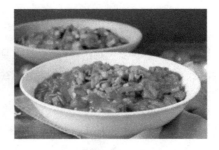

Ever imagined how a Pizza can be turned into soup? Surprise your guests with this unique concoction that combines the flavors of a pizza and delight of your favorite soup.

Ingredients:
- 12 ounce of sliced up chicken sausage
- 4 ounce of uncured pepperoni
- One can of 25 ounces marinara
- One can of 14.5-ounce fire roasted tomatoes
- One diced up a large onion
- 16 ounce of sliced mushroom
- One can of 3 ounces sliced up black olives
- One tablespoon of dried oregano
- One teaspoon of garlic powder
- ½ a teaspoon of salt

Preparation:

1) Take sizeable sized saucepan and toss in the pepperoni, sausage, marinara, onions, tomatoes, mushroom, oregano, olives, salt and garlic powder

2) Cook the mixture for 30 minutes over medium level heat and soften the mushroom and onions

3) Serve hot

39. Spicy Pumpkin Paleo Chili

(Prepping time: 10 minutes\ Cooking time: 15 minutes |For five servings)

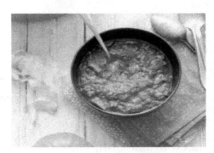

Hate pumpkins but crave for a little spice in your love? This recipe will give you the perfect blend of pumpkin with just the right amount of spicy goodness to satisfy the dragon in you.

Ingredients:

- 3 cups of chopped up yellow onion
- Eight cloves of chopped up garlic
- 1 pound of ground turkey
- Two can of 15-ounce fire roasted tomato
- 2 cups of pumpkin puree
- 1 cup of chicken broth
- Two tablespoon of honey
- Four teaspoon of chili spice
- One teaspoon of ground cinnamon
- One teaspoon of sea salt

Preparation:

1) Take a large sized pot and Sautee your onion and garlic in poured down coconut oil for about 5 minutes

2) Toss in the ground turkey and break it up using your spatula then cook for another 5 minutes

3) Toss in the rest of the ingredients listed and bring it to simmer after mixing

4) Simmer for about 15 minutes without a lid

5) Pour in the chicken broth 6) Serve with a chunk of big salad

40. Tangy Creamy Basil and Tomato Chicken
(Prepping time: 10 minutes\ Cooking time: 20 minutes |For four servings)

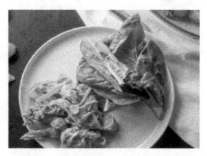

This recipe will give you the perfect meal if you are looking for something a little bit tangy but has the benefits of green vegetables and protein punch of chicken.

Ingredients:
- 1 pound of boneless and skinless chicken breast
- ½ a yellow onion
- One teaspoon of coconut oil
- Three cloves of garlic
- Two tablespoon of sunflower seeds
- One tablespoon of nutritional yeast
- One package of basil
- One tablespoon of avocado oil
- Salt as needed
- Pepper as needed
- ½ a cup of coconut milk
- ½ a teaspoon of arrowroot powder

- 1/3 cup of cold water
- 1 cup of sliced up cherry tomatoes

Preparation:

1) Heat up your coconut oil over a large-sized skillet at medium-high heat and sizzle it

2) Slice up your onion into fine strips and toss them in the heating pan to cook it translucent

3) Once entirely translucent, throw in the chicken to your pan and bake for 12 minutes and flip the chicken only to cook for another 13 minutes

4) In the meantime, take a plate and toss in the garlic in a food processor bowl to finely mince it using the processor

5) Toss in the sunflower seed and pulse it yet again

6) Toss in the nutritional yeast, some salt and just a dash of pepper

7) Pulse until fully minced

8) Take a small bowl and whisk up your arrowroot powder in a water

9) Pour in the coconut milk and whist the pest mixture previously made in

10) Pour the sauce into the chicken skillet and bring it to a delicate simmer

11) Add the sliced cherry tomatoes and allow them to simmer for a while longer, like 1-2 minutes then serve hot

41. Amazing Ground Turkey and Spinach Stuffed Mushroom

(Prepping time: 10 minutes\ Cooking time: 15 minutes |For two servings)

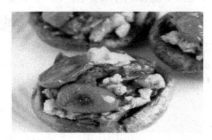

Ground up your Turkey and stuff them in Portobello Mushrooms to create something truly delicious that is both meaty and healthy with the power of Popeye's Spinach.

Ingredients:
- Two teaspoon of coconut oil
- Six large Portobello mushroom with their caps cleared and gills removed.
- 1 diced up a small onion
- ½ a pound of ground turkey
- A handful of baby spinach leaves
- 6-8 grape tomatoes sliced up
- Slat as needed
- Pepper as needed

Preparation:

1) Take a large sized skillet and place it over medium-high heat

2) Toss in 2 teaspoons of coconut oil to melt them and toss your mushroom into the skillet only to cook for minutes until softened

3) Flip them halfway through and place aside

4) In the same skillet, stir in the onion and sauté it until tender which take no more than 3 minutes

5) After a while throw in the ground turkey to the pan and break it up into small pieces using a spatula

6) Cook it further and season with some pepper and salt

7) Once cooked, remove the heat and toss in the baby spinach and allow them to wilt 8) Take a small spoon and scoop up the filling inside the caps of mushroom and top it with some grape tomatoes only to serve hot!

42. Rare Shepherd's Pie with Cauliflower Topping
(Prepping time: 30 minutes\ Cooking time: 30 minutes |For 4-6 servings)

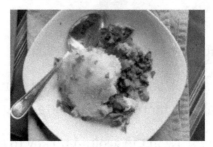

Indeed a Shepherd pie isn't something g that you see every day. But a Shepherd's Pie covered up with Cauliflower? Now that's crazy!

Ingredients:

- One head of cauliflower chopped up into florets
- Four tablespoon of ghee
- 1 diced up a small onion
- 2 diced up celery ribs
- Two minced up garlic cloves
- 1 pound of ground beef
- ¼ -1/2 a cup of homemade beef broth
- One tablespoon of homemade ketchup
- Two tablespoon of chopped up parsley
- Salt as needed
- Pepper as needed

Preparation:

1) Start off by preheating your oven to a temperature of 400 degrees Fahrenheit and grease up about 2-3 quart casserole dish for the future

2) Take a large sized pot and steam your cauliflower until fully softened

3) Heat up two tablespoons of fat in a large sized skillet at medium-high level heat and toss in the onion, celery, garlic, and carrot and cook it until finely softened. Should not take more than 5 minutes

4) Toss in the ground meat and cook it until thoroughly browned. Keep the mixture wet by adding in beef broth

5) Add the ketchup, parsley and season it with pepper and salt and let it simmer while you prepare your cauliflower

6) For the topping, you are going to drain up your cooked cauliflower and mash them with a blender until very smooth

7) Toss in about two tablespoons of fat and season with pepper and salt

8) For the assembling part, take your dish and spread the meat mixture on the bottom 9) Top the meat mixture with cauliflower mixture and smooth with spoon once again covering it with shredded cheese

10) Bake for about 30 minutes and serve warm once when the top is browned up

43. World's Easiest Sweet and Sour Pork Chop
(Prepping time: 5 minutes\ Cooking time: 10 minutes |For four servings)

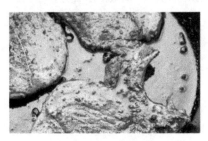

Making Pork Chop to the perfect consistency might seem a little awkward, but don't be afraid! With this recipe, you will be able to cook the ideal Pork chop in no time even if you are a beginner!

Ingredients: For the recipe

- Four pieces of pork chops with the bone still intact
- One teaspoon of fine grain salt
- 1/8 teaspoon of ground black pepper
- Two tablespoon of butter

For the glaze

- Two tablespoon of balsamic vinegar
- Two tablespoon of honey
- Two minced up garlic clove
- ½ a teaspoon of dried rosemary
- ½ a teaspoon of dried oregano

- Pinch of red pepper flakes as needed

Preparation:
1. The first step is to preheat your oven to a temperature of 400 degrees Fahrenheit and place a rack in the middle section
2. Season up your pork with pepper and salt and set it aside
3. Take a large sized iron skillet and melt your butter over over medium-high heat
4. While sizzling, toss in the seasoned pork chops and sear them until both sides are golden. Making sure to go for 2 minutes cooking for each side
5. Place the processed pork in your oven and roast for 6 minutes
6. While it is roasted, go ahead and prepare your glaze by taking a small saucepan and tossing in all of the listed ingredients and bringing it to a boil at medium-high heat
7. Then reduce the temperature and simmer it for 5 minutes
8. Remove the pork from the oven and serve by pouring in the glaze all over them.
9. Bake for another 4 minutes in the oven and serve hot!

44. Extravagant Graham Crackers

(Prepping time: 15 minutes\ Cooking time: 30 minutes |For 4-6 servings)

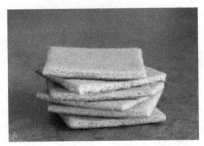

Graham Crackers are incredibly healthy we all know it. But getting Graham Crackers from the market might be tough, primarily Paleo suitable ones. With this recipe, you will easily be able to make Graham Crackers that are perfect for our Paleo Diet.

Ingredients:
- 2 cups of ¼ full almond flour
- One teaspoon of baking powder
- One teaspoon of ground cinnamon
- ½ a teaspoon of fine sea salt
- One large sized egg
- Two tablespoon of melted coconut oil
- Two tablespoon of pure maple syrup

Preparation:

1) Take a large sized bowl and whisk in everything including the baking powder, almond meal, salt and cinnamon

2) Toss in the egg, maple syrup, and coconut oil and keep stirring it until it has blended itself to an excellent dough with strong adhesion

3) Cover up your bowl and let it chill for 30 minutes

4) Preheat your oven to a temperature 325 degree Fahrenheit and line it up a large cookie sheet with parchment paper

5) Top it off with another parchment paper sheet and use a rolling pin to roll the dough to 1/8 inch thickness

6) Take a pizza cutter and cut out 2.5-inch squares and transfer them to the prepared sheet

7) Bake in your oven for about 15 minutes until nicely browned

8) Cool for 5 minutes and server the crunchy delights.

45. Wholly Appetizing Mango Chia Seed Pudding

(Prepping time: 10 minutes\ Cooking time: 60 minutes |For four servings)

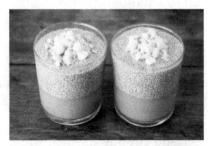

Why not end the day with something chilly? Make up a whole cup of Mango Chia Seed Pudding! This double layer Pudding will wrap up your thirst and satisfy hunger as well.

Ingredients:
- One whole mango completely peeled up and pureed
- One full cup of 250ml coconut milk
- 3 tablespoon of chia seed

Preparation:

1) This is a very straightforward recipe which only requires you to combine all of the mentioned ingredients in a bowl and let it chill for about an hour.

2) Once relaxed, just take it out and serve!

46. Chocolaty Cocoa Mousse

(Prepping time: 10 minutes\ Cooking time: nil |For four servings)

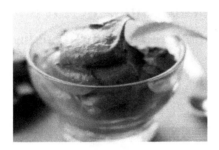

If you have a midnight Chocolate Mousse craving, then this recipe will satisfy your need. In just a few minutes, you will be able to batch up this fine mousse.

Ingredients:
- Coconut cream scraped from the upper side of 2 13.5 ounce chilled cans of full-fat coconut milk
- Four tablespoon of cocoa
- Three tablespoon of honey
- One teaspoon of vanilla extract

Preparation:

1) The first step is to open up your cans and scoop out the thick coconut cream and toss them to a large bowl

2) In that bowl, throw in the honey, cocoa, vanilla extract and beat using your mixer starting from low going all the way to medium until a nice foam appears

3) Divide the mixtures into even ramekins and chill those to your desired level of cold

47. Exquisite Pumpkin Nut Butter Cup
(Prepping time: 120 minutes\ Cooking time: nil |For four servings)

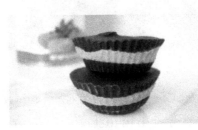

Who says muffin are banned in Paleo? This recipe will allow you to create exquisitely delicious Pumpkin Nut Butter Cups with multiple layers of goodness. One with chocolate and the other with pumpkin puree!

Ingredients: For Filing

- ½ a cup of organic pumpkin puree
- 1/2a cup of homemade almond butter
- Two tablespoon of organic maple syrup
- Four tablespoon of organic coconut oil
- ¼ teaspoon of organic ground nutmeg
- ¼ teaspoon of organic ground ginger
- One teaspoon of organic ground cinnamon
- 1/8 teaspoon of organic ground clove
- Two teaspoon of natural vanilla extract

  For Topping

- 1 cup of organic raw cacao powder
- Four tablespoon of organic maple syrup
- 1 cup of organic coconut oil

Preparation:

1) Firstly you are going to need to make the pumpkin filling, to do this take a medium-sized bowl and pour in all of the ingredients listed under pumpkin filling and mix them until creamy

2) For the chocolate topping, make another bowl and combine in all of the ingredients listed under chocolate topping until smooth and creamy

3) Then, make a muffin cup and fill about 1/3 of it with chocolate topping 4) Keep in freezer and chill for 15 minutes

5) Fill another 1/3 with pumpkin filling

6) And finally, fill the last part with another layer of chocolate mix

7) Put in freezer and chill for 2 hours

8) Store and take out to eat when desired.

48. Tender Chocolate Silk Pie

(Prepping time: 90 minutes\ Cooking time: nil |For 16 servings)

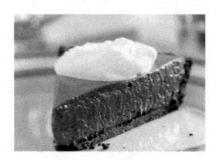

This is a relatively simple recipe that will teach you how to bake up your very own Chocolate Silk Pie. A delightful layer of chocolate cake that is mixed with healthy boost of Avocados.

Ingredients:
- 8 ounce of Dark Chocolate
- ¼ cup of extra virgin olive oil
- Two ripe Avocados
- 1 cup of coconut sugar
- 1 and a ½ cup of cocoa powder
- 1 cup of heavy cream
- One tablespoon of vanilla
- ½ a teaspoon of espresso powder
- Just a pinch of salt

Preparation:

1) The first step here is to take a pan and toss in the dark chocolate in coconut oil at medium heat

2) Once done, let the chocolate cool at room temperature

3) Then scoop out some avocado meat and place them in a mixing bowl

4) Add the chocolate coconut mixture to the very pan alongside cocoa powder and sugar

5) Whip up the mix on medium speed using a mixer for about 2-3 minutes

6) Toss in the extract, cream, salt, and espresso and whip it again on medium high to high speed for approximately 5 minutes until thoroughly fluffy

7) Divide the batter into pie crust portions and chill them for a few hours 8) Serve with whipped cream!

49. Turkey Lettuce Wrap Tacos

You might miss the crunch of those carbohydrate filled tacos, but this recipe calls for a paleo transformation that cuts out the carb filled shell entirely in favor of a crunchy crust made of lettuce! These turkey lettuce wraps are loaded with meat, even while stocking up on plenty of tasty veggies, herbs, and spices. So forget all about stopping at Taco Bell after work! Just go home and make yourself some paleo friendly Turkey Lettuce Wrap Tacos! You are going to love it!

Here are the exact ingredients:
- One teaspoon of olive oil
- One teaspoon of fresh, minced garlic
- 1 cup of diced jalapeno's (For that extra kick!"
- One teaspoon of cumin
- ¼ teaspoon cayenne pepper
- 2 pounds ground turkey

½ a teaspoon of salt
- 1 cup of diced green onions
- 1 cup of freshly chopped cilantro
- One teaspoon of lime juice
- Two heads of romaine lettuce

1. Pour your olive oil into your frying pan and set your burner to high. Next, go ahead and toss in your minced garlic, and add your diced jalapenos and let the contents of the pan cook for a couple of minutes.
2. You can then add your teaspoons of cumin, cayenne pepper, and allow them to cook together for another minute or so.
3. After this, add in your 2 pounds of turkey, salting with you ½ teaspoon of salt, letting the turkey cook until it turns brown.
4. While your turkey is browning, get out your cutting board and use it to dice up your green onions.
5. Set these onions to the side for the moment and pick up your fresh cilantro, wash it and then chop it into small pieces.
6. Now stir in your cilantro with the rest of the ingredients. Now take your romaine lettuce head and cut out the core.
7. Get rid of the rougher outer layers, before extracting the fresh lettuce underneath.
8. Try to peel large swaths of lettuce off of the lettuce head intact, so that you can use it hold your taco ingredients.
9. Just take a spoon and scoop up your turkey mixture right into the lettuce and fold it into the shape of a taco! Your delicious Turkey Lettuce Wrap Tacos are now ready for their midday meal debut!

50. Shredded Chicken Breasts with freshly chopped Thyme

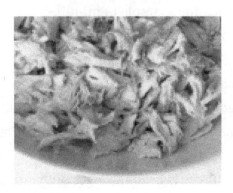

It's healthy, it's delicious, and its paleo! There is nothing in this recipe that our hunter-gatherer ancestors couldn't have grabbed up in the wilderness. It consists of fresh chicken, with fennel seeds, mint, and a bit of thyme. Shredded chicken breasts, with just a dash of freshly chopped thyme, will make just about anyone happy! This dish will make your midday meal something to look forward to!

Here are the exact ingredients:
- One lean chicken breast
- ¼ cup of fennel seeds
- Three tablespoons of finely chopped thyme
- Five tablespoons of olive oil
- ¼ cup of roughly torn mint
- One lemon wedge

1. Fill a medium sized pan up with water and place it on the burner, set at medium heat.
2. With war water nearing the boiling point, you can then drop your lean chicken breast into the pan.
3. Let this chicken boil for about 5 minutes before removing it from the pan. Place the chicken on a clean cutting board and let it cool down for a few moments.
4. After cooling, start cutting the meat up with a knife until it is shredded into small pieces; dump these pieces into a medium mixing bowl.
5. Next, add your fennel seeds, thyme, olive oil, and mix them with your shredded chicken, making sure that the chicken gets well marinated with all of the ingredients.
6. Once marinated adequately like this, you can take out as much as you would like to eat and place it on a plate for consumption.
7. As a finishing touch, slice off yourself a lemon wedge so you can sprinkle lemon juice on the shredded chicken making this paleo meal even more delicious than it already is.

51. Paleo Stir Fried Fajita's

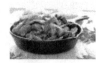

There is nothing quite like some good stir fry for your midday meal. This dish also combines some Latin flavor and spice for a much-needed kick for your midday paleo routine. So mark your calendar for a day that you can enjoy yourself this deliciously paleo, stir-fried fajita's!

Here are the exact ingredients:
- 3 pounds of beef steak
- 1 cup of olive oil
- ½ cup of crushed garlic
- ¼ cup of lime juice
- ¼ cup chili powder
- ¼ cup cumin
- ½ cup red bell pepper, chopped
- ½ cup yellow bell pepper, cut
- ½ cup chopped onion
- One diced Roma tomato
- ¼ cup cilantro, chopped

1. First, put your 3 pounds of beef in a glass container. Next, take out a separate plastic container and add precisely

one half of your cup of olive oil, save the rest for later, you will need it.

2. Follow this than by adding your ½ cup of crushed garlic, ¼ cup of lime juice, ¼ cup of chili powder, and your ¼ cup of cumin.

3. Stir these together well before pouring the entire contents of the container out on top of your beef in the glass cooking pan.

4. Now put your glass cooking pan in the refrigerator and let it soak up the flavor of all the ingredients for 2 hours in the fridge.

5. Now take that other half of your olive oil that you saved and dump it into a pan and let it cook over medium heat.

6. After this take out your glass container and drop your marinated beef steak into the pot.

7. Next, add your onions, diced tomatoes, and peppers and let the mixture cook for a few minutes while you stir the contents.

8. Turn off your burner and add your chopped cilantro as a finishing touch. Your Paleo Stir Fried Fajita's are now ready for consumption!

52. Turkey Paleo Skewers

Meat on a stick? This meal is pretty straightforward and self-explanatory, and even a cave dweller could do it! Don't worry about getting a little bit messy with this recipe, it's well worth it!

Here are the exact ingredients:
- Five wooden skewers
- One lean turkey breast
- Two tablespoons of olive oil
- Two tablespoons of chopped sage
- Two tablespoons of vinegar

1. First, take your olive oil and vinegar and mix them well in a mixing bowl. Now set this mixture to the side and take out a clean cutting board and use it to chop up your thawed turkey breast. Add this chopped turkey breast to the mixing bowl of vinegar and oil and let it marinate in the mix for a few moments before putting a plastic covering over it and storing it in your refrigerator.
2. Let it stay in the fridge for a few hours, taking it out just to shift the ingredients around in the bowl every so often.

3. After sitting in your refrigerator for a few hours, take the dish out, and using wooden skewers, skewer the meat onto the wooden sticks.
4. You can then cook them over an open flame such as a campfire, or over a grill making for some tasty Turkey Paleo Skewers right in the middle of your day.

53. Paleo Slow Cooked Chicken

This is a hearty midday meal right out of the Paleolithic past—that is—if the Paleolithic era had slow cookers! Because in this recipe you will find delicious chicken and juicy onions, seasoned to perfection with herbs and spices, just one slow-cooked meal away from you! Just toss your chicken in the pot and get ready for a great way to kick off your midday!

Here are the exact ingredients:
- Two lean chicken breasts
- 1 cup chopped onion
- ¼ cup paprika
- ¼ cup cayenne pepper
- ¼ cup black pepper
- ¼ cup poultry seasoning
- ¼ cup garlic powder

1. Get your slow cooker out and set it on high heat, before dropping your cup of chopped onions down to the bottom of the stove.
2. After you have done this, move on to blend your spices in a medium-sized mixing bowl.
3. Add your paprika, cayenne pepper, black pepper, and poultry seasoning together and mix them well.
4. Then take these mixed spices and pour them over your chicken breasts.
5. Put these now newly spiced up chicken breasts and put them right on top of the onions lining the bottom of your slow cooker.
6. You can now put the lid on your stove and begin the 4 to 5-hour process of cooking up this paleo midday meal.
7. It isn't necessary to add any water or anything like that since your chicken breasts should have enough natural juice inside of them already. Enjoy!
8. The last meal of the day should be able to sustain you through the rest of the night, without breaking your diet.
9. Many of us have self-control issues when we come home from a long day of work, and end up overeating for our evening meal.
10. To avoid this; merely plan it out. Take a look at these recipes and suppertime meal plans so that you can do just that!

54. Meaty Eggplant Meal

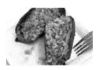

Eggplant is one of my favorite veggies, and when it is served with lean meat and fresh garlic, it is even better. This meal is filling without breaking the carbohydrate bank account, and the ingredients are so simple they firmly classify as Paleolithic in their makeup. And the taste of lean hamburger meat roasted with onions and tomatoes just can't be beaten! Find a place for this great recipe, at the end of your busy day.

Here are the exact ingredients:
- ½ pound of lean hamburger
- ¼ cup chopped onions
- ¼ cup of tomato paste
- ¼ cup diced tomatoes
- One eggplant
- 2 cups of lettuce

1. The first thing you should do is cut your eggplant in half lengthwise.
2. Put this eggplant in a baking pan and let it cook in the oven for about 10 minutes at 400 degrees Fahrenheit.
3. While your eggplant is cooking take your hamburger and place it in a frying pan on high heat, add your cup of

chopped onions and begin stirring it together vigorously as it melts.

4. Next, add your tomato paste and your ¼ cup of diced tomatoes and stir these in as well.
5. Now turn your burner down to low heat and let the mixture cook for another 10 minutes.
6. Turn off your burner and get out a large plate, spread out your lettuce on this plate and set it down on your counter.
7. With your salad in place, take your cooked eggplant out of the oven and place it on top of the plate of salad.
8. After you have done this, you can then pour your hamburger, tomato, and onion mixture out of your frying pan and drizzle it out on top of the lettuce and eggplant.
9. This meal is a delicious and satisfying way to have a supper that's straight out of the Stone Age.

55. Paleo Salmon and Chanterelle Mushroom

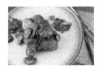

This mushroom and salmon fish dish would have been a real treat back in the Stone Age, and makes for a great supper today! Just look at this grilled fish and delicious mushroom combo! And nothing brings out the flavor like white wine! I hope you enjoy this Paleolithic dish, because I know I do!

Here are the exact ingredients:

- Three salmon filets
- 1 cup chopped chanterelle mushrooms
- ½ cup of olive oil
- ¼ cup of white wine
- ½ cup thyme leaves
- ¼ cup garlic
- ¼ cup butter

1. Set your grill to medium-high, and stretch your salmon filets out on the restaurant.
2. Take a marinating brush and rub some olive oil directly onto your salmon filets.
3. Let your salmon cook. And while your salmon is cooking on the grill (or as the Australians like to call it "the Barbie"), get out a medium-sized frying pan and place it on your stove with the burner set to medium.
4. To this pan, you will add your mushrooms, garlic, butter, thyme leaves, white wine, and the rest of your olive oil.
5. Let these cook for about 3 minutes while you stir the contents vigorously. Once cooked put your mushroom and thyme leaves the mixture on a plate and add your salmon fillets to the dish.
6. Your Stone Age Supper is now ready to eat!

56. Yellow Peppers, Broccoli Rabe, and Poached Egg

This paleo dinner dish takes the best of all natural broccoli, peppers, and eggs, and makes them into a super supper for any era! The veggies are cooked in succulently soft, and the eggs just melt in your mouth! Supper is a sight to see with this Stone Age recipe!

Here are the exact ingredients:
- ½ cup chopped broccoli rabe
- ½ cup chopped yellow sweet peppers
- ¼ cup of olive oil
- Three eggs

1. Put a pan of water on your stove and set the heat on high. Drop your half cup of chopped broccoli rabe into the pan and let it boil for about 5 minutes.
2. After this, drain the pot of water and make your broccoli lose some of its heat. Next, add your ¼ cup of olive oil and your ½ cup of chopped yellow sweet peppers.
3. Now, put the burner on medium heat and as you stir the mixture, let the entire contents of the pan cook for another 5 minutes.

4. Turn the burner off and let the materials of your pan absorb the residual heat.
5. Setting these ingredients to the side for the moment, get out a medium-sized mixing bowl and break your three eggs open, dropping the egg's contents inside the container.
6. Cover the pan with cling film and seal the pot with the material. Flip the bowl upside down letting the eggs move to the surface of the film.
7. Lift the container up and close the film up over the eggs, allowing it seal up around them like a plastic bag.
8. Boil the eggs while they are nestled in this film, this will poach your paleo eggs.
9. Now merely throw your poached eggs, yellow peppers, and broccoli rabe on a plate, and this Stone Age supper is ready to eat!

57. Shiitake Meat Loaf

Everyone likes a little meatloaf right? Well, what about some paleo meatloaf? Cooked in abundant olive oil, roasted with mushrooms and tomatoes, while being marinated in onion powder, flaxseed, and red wine, this recipe is a suppertime hero. And this shiitake meatloaf blend won't disappoint!

Here are the exact ingredients:

- ½ cup of olive oil
- ¼ cup chopped shiitake mushrooms
- 1 cup diced tomatoes
- 1 pound grass fed beef
- ¼ cup flaxseed
- ¼ cup onion powder
- ¼ cup red wine
- Two eggs

1. First, preheat your oven to 400 degrees. Next, put your half cup of olive oil into a frying pan and put it on a burner set on high heat.
2. After you have done this, you can then add your shiitake mushrooms and tomatoes, and let them cook for a few minutes.
3. Now remove the pan from the burner and let it cool off for a few more minutes.
4. You can now put the contents of the container into a blender and blend it all. Get out a small plastic bowl and add your two eggs, a pound of beef, ¼ cup of flaxseed and ¼ cup of onion powder and mix them.
5. Now dump this mixture into a baking pan. Use a spoon to pat down the surface of the dough uniformly.
6. Next, grab your container of cooked shiitake mushrooms and tomatoes and dump them on top of the meat mixture in the pan.

7. As a finishing touch take your ¼ cup of red wine and lightly pour it over the surface of your baking pan meatloaf mixture.
8. Bake for about an hour and your shiitake meatloaf is finished.

58. Vegetable and Beef Stew Supper

I used to love beefed stew as a kid, but as an adult, the high sodium and carbs haven't always been the best thing for my diet. But the paleo version serves to fix all of that once and for all. Cooked in healthy olive oil, and roasted with paleo-friendly carrots, celery, and squash, this Vegetable and Beef Stew makes for the perfect Stone Age supper!

Here are the exact ingredients:
- ½ cup of olive oil
- 1 pound of cubed chuck steak
- 1 cup chopped onion
- ½ cup chopped garlic
- 1 cup chopped carrots
- 1 cup chopped celery

- ½ cup chopped squash
- 1 cup chicken broth
- ¼ cup oregano
- A dash of ground black pepper

Preparation:
1. First, add your ½ cup of olive oil to a frying pan and set your burner to medium heat.
2. Next, add your pound of cubed steak to the pan and cook the meat until it is thoroughly brown.
3. After you have done this, add your chopped garlic, onion, carrots, celery and squash to the pan and stir them into the mix while they cook with the meat for another few minutes.
4. Now you can pour in your cup of chicken broth, bring the mixture to a boil, put on a lid, set the burner to low heat, and let the contents of the pan soak up the low temperature for the next half hour.
5. Stir regularly during this 30 minute period, and add as much black pepper as you like.
6. Invite some friends because your vegetable and beef stew is ready for supper!

59. Minced Indian Curry

Even though Curry didn't exactly exist in the Paleolithic Era, all of the ingredients that make up this batch did! So let's get ready to make some tremendous minced Indian Curry. If Curry did exist in the Stone Age, it should have tasted like this!

Here are the exact ingredients:
- 1 pound of minced beef
- ½ cup chopped onion
- ½ cup chopped garlic
- ½ cup of olive oil
- 3 cups of chopped cabbage
- 1 cup of chopped eggplant
- ½ cup chopped tomatoes
- ¼ cup of curry

1. To get started, go to your cutting board and begin cutting up your onion, garlic, and a pound of beef.
2. After these are appropriately sliced and diced throw them into a pot and turn the burner on high heat letting the contents cook for about 7 minutes.
3. Turn the burner off and let the contents cool off for a few more minutes before dropping the ingredients into a separate container.
4. Now turn your burner back on high, and add your curry, chopped cabbage, chopped tomatoes, chopped eggplant and your olive oil, and start stirring the contents together.

5. After a few minutes of this take your separate container of the beef, onion, and garlic mixture and dump it back into the pan.
6. Now stir everything together for a few more minutes on high heat. Turn off the burner, let the contents cool, and then serve when ready.

60. Paleo Barbeque Chicken

Whether it's a backyard suppertime barbeque or regular meal in the house, Paleo Barbeque Chicken won't disappoint! With lean chicken breasts cooked in healthy olive oil, and marinated with oregano, chopped garlic, and lemon juice, this Stone Age Supper is the best!

Here are the exact ingredients:
- Three lean chicken breasts (A whole lot of paleo chicken!)
- ½ cup of olive oil
- ½ cup chopped cloves of garlic
- ¼ cup of cumin
- ½ cup of oregano
- ¼ cup lemon juice

1. Mix your garlic, olive oil, paprika, cumin oregano, and lemon juice in a small mixing bowl.

2. With these ingredients adequately mixed take out a clean cutting board and start slicing your chicken breasts into medium sized strips.
3. Take these strips and drop them into your mixing bowl with your other ingredients.
4. With clean hands rub these ingredients onto your chicken breasts, let them sit in the pan for a few more minutes, so that they can further marinate themselves.
5. Next, put some plastic wrap over the mixing bowl and let it sit in your refrigerator for a couple of hours, stirring it occasionally.
6. After your marinated chicken has cooled, take out the container and take it on over to your grill.
7. Set your rack to medium heat and place your chicken strips on top.
8. Let these strips cook for about 15 minutes, or until they are well browned on each side. This is some of the best barbeque chicken you could ever find!

61. Paleo Braised River Trout

At the end of the day, you need something that is both delicious and nutritious to sustain you. These Paleo Braised River Trout do just that! This type of trout is exceptional and is best when you catch it yourself in the wild. But if you don't have access (or time) to do all that, you can find this fish at most health food stores. Just make sure you do your homework, and you too can have your very own Paleo Braised River Trout for supper tonight!

Here are the exact ingredients:

- ¼ cup of olive oil
- 1 cup chopped carrots
- 1 cup chicken broth
- Five river trout fillets
- A dash of black pepper

1. Add your ¼ cup of olive oil to a medium-sized pan and set the burner to high. Next, add your carrots and stir them while they cook.
2. After you have done this, you can add your cup of chicken broth and bring the whole mixture to a boil.
3. Adjust your high heat setting to a lower one and add your fish to the pan. Sprinkle a dash of black pepper on the fish to add just the right amount of extra flavoring.
4. Your Paleo Braised River Trout is now ready to serve and eat.

62. The Prehistoric Beef Tenderloin Roast

Our ancestors were eating like this before anyone knew to write about it! It was quite common for the hunter-gatherers of the past to bag some wild game, roast it over the fire and then eat it with whatever other wild morsels that they found just growing in the wilderness! Just try it, and you will like it! Because this fantastic dish takes grass-fed beef right to the next level! With a whole pound of lean beef, cooked in olive oil marinated in flaxseed oil, chopped parsley, as well as cut garlic and shallots, this recipe makes for a feast from the Stone Age!

Here are the exact ingredients:
- 1 pound of beef steak
- ¼ cup of olive oil
- ½ cup of shiitake mushrooms
- ¼ cup chopped garlic
- ¼ cup chopped shallots
- ¼ cup chopped parsley
- ¼ cup flaxseed oil
- Two large kale leaves

1. To get started to take your beef out of the refrigerator and let it thaw (if it isn't already) and let it sit out for about half of an hour.
2. While your meat is melting set your oven to about 375 degrees, to preheat. Next, add your ¼ cup of olive oil to the pan over a burner set on high.
3. Toss in your mushrooms and vigorously stir them over the heat, and cook them for about ten minutes.
4. After the ten minutes are up, take your mushrooms out of the pan and set them to the side.
5. Now put your pan back on the burner, set it to high heat, and put your pound of beef steak in the pan.
6. In this step in the process, you are just going to sear each side of the beefsteak in the high heat for about 5 minutes on each side, or until brown.
7. After doing this, take the meat out of the pan and put it in a baking pan in your already preheated oven.
8. And while your chicken is cooking, gauge the progress by inserting a meat thermometer into the steak.
9. Just to give you an idea of what to look for; 160 degrees signifies steak that is well done, 140 degrees is medium, 130 degrees is medium rare (that hits the spot!), and 120 degrees is rare.
10. As anyone who has ever gone to their local steakhouse no doubt knows, everyone has a different idea of what a good steak is.
11. Some like their steaks well done and others like them medium rare, just remember, the more undercooked your

meat is, the more at risk you may be for pathogens in the beef such as e coli and salmonella.

12. I like a medium rare steak as much as anyone else—but it is true—the less you cook your steaks, the more risk you may be taking.

13. So going with the happy medium, try to cook your meat until it is medium or well done.

14. After your chicken is cooked merely add in your chopped shallots, chopped parsley, chopped garlic, and ¼ cup of flaxseed oil and this Prehistoric Beef Tenderloin is ready for business!

Salads

63. Paleo Chili with Turkey

This chili may be a leftover from the Paleolithic Era, but it tastes just as good as any other chili I've ever had! This dish works well because it substitutes the typical ingredient in most chilies—beans—with more paleo friendly ingredients such as carrots and bell peppers. It still tastes great, and you don't have to worry about the consequences of wrecking your diet (or facing the <u>other</u> implications that beans often bring)! Ground turkey garnished with carrots, onions, bell peppers, and thyme makes for quite a wonderful time!

Here are the exact ingredients:
- ½ pound of ground turkey
- ¼ cup of olive oil
- ½ cup chopped onions
- ½ cup chopped carrots
- ½ cup chopped red bell peppers
- ½ cup chopped yellow bell peppers
- ¼ cup chopped thyme
- ¼ cup of ground cumin
- ½ cup of paprika

- ¼ cup of chili flakes
- One can of diced tomatoes
- ¼ cup of lemon juice

1. First, boil your ground turkey on high heat for about 15 minutes. Turn the burner off and put this pan to the side.
2. Take out another pan and put it on medium heat. In this pan go ahead and add your bell peppers, carrots, garlic, and onions to the pan.
3. Let these ingredients cook for just a few minutes before adding your cumin, thyme, paprika, and chili flakes to the mix.
4. Now take a wooden spoon and vigorously whisk these ingredients together for a couple of minutes.
5. Turn your burner to low heat, and let the ingredients simmer while you add your ground turkey to the pan.
6. Cook the entire contents of the container for another 10 minutes before serving.

64. Paleo Salmon Caesar Salad

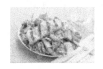

Fresh Caesar salad is delicious, and this paleo blend is even better! The Omega 3s in particular that are found in this dish makes for a significant part of a paleo diet. A good dose of Omega 3 can help decrease your risk for cardiovascular disease, prevent the development of arthritis and even cure depression, all great reasons to have a good Caesar salad!

Here are the exact ingredients:

- Three salmon fillets
- ¼ cup of olive oil
- One head of chopped romaine lettuce
- ½ cup chopped onion
- ¼ cup of flaxseed oil
- ¼ cup of crushed garlic
- ¼ cup of mustard seed
- ¼ cup of lemon juice
- A dash of black pepper

1. Take a cooking brush and use it to drench your salmon fillets with your olive oil.
2. Put them into a baking pan and broil in the oven for about 10 minutes. After which take the salmon out and set it aside.
3. Now take out a mixing bowl, add your lettuce and chopped onion, and mix in your flaxseed oil, mustard seed, garlic, and lemon juice.
4. Once you have stirred these together, put your salmon on top of it and your Paleo Salmon Caesar Salad.

65. Chicken Salad and Walnuts

This salad will fill you up and not bust your paleo dietary budget! All you need is one lean chicken breast, some arugula leaves, a bit of seasoning and some walnuts and your chicken salad is complete!

Here are the exact ingredients:
- One lean chicken breast
- ¼ cup of Cajun chicken seasoning
- ¼ cup chopped walnuts
- 2 cups of arugula leaves
- One green apple, sliced and diced
- ¼ cup of lemon juice
- ¼ cup of honey
- ¼ cup of olive oil
- ¼ cup of vinegar

1. Set your oven to 400 degrees. Get out an oven tray and place some safe baking paper down at the bottom of it.
2. Next, get out your cutting board and cut up your chicken breast into finely chopped pieces.
3. Put your freshly diced chicken into a plastic bowl, from here; begin drizzling your ¼ cup of Cajun chicken seasoning onto your diced chicken.

4. After you have done, this put your chicken pieces and put them on your oven tray, and place the plate into the oven. Let's these cook for at least 10 minutes.
5. With your chicken in the oven, now you can turn to the preparation of the rest of your ingredients.
6. First, put your ¼ cup of chopped walnuts, put them in a pan, and set the burner to high.
7. Now just let these nuts roast until they turn brown, occasionally stirring them. After this, take out your arugula leaves, your sliced and diced apples, your ¼ cup of honey, ¼ cup of lemon juice, ¼ cup of olive oil, and your ¼ cup of vinegar and put them in a small mixing bowl.
8. Stir the contents of your container together before dumping the contents onto a large plate; this will constitute the salad of your <u>chicken salad</u>.
9. Just take your chopped chicken out of the oven and put it right on top of this paleo-terrific plate of salad!

66. Leftover Hash

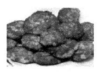

Just because it's leftover doesn't mean it's not going to be good! Take this leftover hash as a prime example! All you got to do is take a little bit of beef and mix up with some sweet potato, chopped onions, and tomato sauce and you are in for a delicious leftover from the Paleolithic Era!

Here are the exact ingredients:
- 1 cup chopped sweet potato
- ½ cup chopped onion
- ¼ pound of beef or hamburger leftovers
- ½ cup tomato sauce
- ¼ cup of coconut oil

1. Get started on the main component of your leftover hash first; the sweet potato.
2. Chop this sweet potato up into small pieces. Next, chop up your onion, until you have about half a cup.
3. After that, place a large saucepan on medium heat and add your coconut oil to the pan.
4. Let this heat up for about 30 seconds before adding your sweet potatoes, onions, tomato sauce and of course, your ¼ of a pound of leftover beef or hamburger.

5. Stir this mixture together, let it cook for about 5 minutes, and these leftovers from the Stone Age are complete!

67. Artichoke Heart Salad

You can eat your heart on this salad because this is a hefty recipe that works well for any day of your 30-day challenge!

Here are the exact ingredients:
- 1 cup of chopped artichoke hearts
- 1 cup chopped red bell pepper
- 1 cup chopped onion
- ½ cup of lemon juice
- ¼ cup of olive oil
- ¼ cup of pepper
- ¼ cup of salt
- ½ cup chopped avocado

1. First, take your cup of chopped artichoke hearts, your cup of chopped onion, your cup of chopped red bell pepper, your ½ cup of lemon juice, and your ¼ cup of olive oil and mix it all together thoroughly in a small bowl.
2. Now sprinkle your ¼ cup of pepper and your ¼ cup of salt on top of the mixture.
3. Finally, add your ½ cup of chopped avocado on top, and your Artichoke Heart Salad is ready to go.
4. This is one of the best paleo recipes you could come by.

68. Cucumber Salad

Crunchy cucumbers and tasty blueberries come together to make a real treat. This salad is healthy, satisfying, and a significant part of the paleo diet.

Here are the exact ingredients:

- Two cucumbers
- ½ cup of chopped blueberries
- ½ cup of olive oil
- ¼ cup of vinegar
- ¼ cup of feta cheese

1. To get started on this paleo recipe you need to take your cucumbers, completely peel them and slice them in half lengthwise.
2. And then cut these slices in half one more time.
3. Add these slices to a large mixing bowl and add your ½ cup of chopped blueberries, your ½ cup of olive oil, your ¼ cup of vinegar, and your ¼ cup of feta cheese.
4. Stir these ingredients together well and serve.

69. Spinach Salad

This Spinach Salad comes complete with chopped strawberries, garlic, vinegar, and olive oil. This is a great salad for the paleo diet; or any other diet for that matter!

Here are the exact ingredients:
- 1 cup chopped strawberries
- ½ cup of olive oil
- ½ cup of vinegar
- ½ cup chopped garlic
- ½ cup of poppy seeds
- ¼ cup of black pepper

1. Add your cup of chopped strawberries, your ½ cup of olive oil, your ½ cup of vinegar, your ½ cup of chopped garlic, your ½ cup of poppy seeds, and your ¼ cup of black pepper to a medium-sized mixing bowl.
2. Thoroughly combine these ingredients and your Spinach Salad is ready to go!

70. Paleo Cucumber Salad

Another great salad for your 30-Day Paleo Challenge! Cucumber, tomatoes, chopped dill and cider vinegar come together like never before!

Here are the exact ingredients:
- 1 cup of chopped cucumber
- 1 cup chopped tomatoes
- ¼ cup of apple cider vinegar
- ¼ cup chopped dill

1. For this recipe, it's easy. All you have to do is add all of your ingredients together in a large mixing bowl and stir well.
2. Once you have done this, you just need to cool the components down a bit by leaving them in your fridge to chill for a couple of hours.
3. This will ensure that the veggies are all excellent and crisp when you serve them.
4. So just mix it all in a bowl, put it in your refrigerator to chill, and this paleolithic recipe is complete!

Paleo Desserts

71. Baked Paleo Apple Desert

As good as an old-fashioned apple pie, these Baked Paleo Apples are just as tasty even without the heavily processed gluten-filled crust of typical apple based deserts. So forget all about that apple pie and give this paleo dessert recipe a try!

Here are the exact ingredients:
- ¼ cup of raisins
- ¼ cup raw walnuts
- ¼ cup cinnamon
- 1 bowl of chopped apples
- ½ cup of water

1. First, set your oven to 400 degrees. Next, take your ¼ cup of raisins, ¼ cup of walnuts, ¼ cup of cinnamon, and mix them in a medium-sized mixing bowl.
2. Now transfer these ingredients to a glass baking pan, and add your cup of chopped apples to the mix as well.

3. Add your ½ cup of water and thoroughly mix your ingredients.

4. Put this mixture in the oven and let it cook for about a half hour.

5. After which your baked paleo apple dessert is ready to serve.

72. Caveman Crème and Strawberries

This dessert is a classic with a paleo twist. Fresh strawberries served without the excess of sweet sugary additives that accompany them. This dish takes out those nonpaleo elements and transforms it into something truly magnificent! If you need a pick me up during your 30 Day Paleo Challenge, give this Caveman Crème and Strawberries recipe a look over!

Here are the exact ingredients:
- 2 cups strawberries, sliced
- ¼ cup of vanilla extract
- ¼ cup of coconut milk

1. This recipe requires some special preparation, so you are going to have to put a whisk and a copper bowl up inside your freezer to chill them for about 25 minutes.

2. Now take out another bowl and add your vanilla extract and strawberries, stir these together before covering them and putting them in the fridge.
3. Next, add your coconut milk to the other bowl that you left in the refrigerator for 25 minutes, and then take your whisk and use it to stir the coconut milk, letting it thicken.
4. This is all you have to do to stiffen your crème. Now take your other bowl and dump your strawberries and vanilla into your thickened crème mixture.
5. Your Caveman Crème and Strawberries are now ready to eat.

73. Paleo Banana Bonanza

Banana's are a fruit to be reckoned with on the paleo diet. One of the great things about bananas is the fact that they are so versatile. And with the help of a few key ingredients—as shown in this recipe—you can make a dessert that everyone will like. Its sweet and it's crunchy, and it's altogether delicious. You don't even have to be a caveman to enjoy this Paleo Banana Bonanza.

Here are the exact ingredients:
- Two large, ripened bananas
- ¼ of a cup of vanilla extract
- ¼ cup of ginger

- ¼ cup of allspice
- ¼ cup of pecans

---

1. This dessert takes the cake (no pun intended). This simple banana recipe makes for a great paleo treat loaded with potassium!
2. To get started, cut your bananas vertically and then put them in a small container.
3. Next, place the bananas face down on a piece of paper wax, before putting them in the freezer and letting them cool down for about half an hour.
4. After this take the bananas out and drizzle your ginger, allspice, pecans, and nutmeg on top of the bananas.
5. Now you can indeed have yourself a Paleo Banana Bonanza!

74. Mango Margarita

Smooth, crisp, and refreshing! This Mango Margarita mix bypasses the corn syrup or other processed sweet drinks, and gives you an even better paleo alternative! There is just nothing better after a hot summer day than a nice fresh round of Mango Margaritas!

Here are the exact ingredients:

- 1 cup of water
- 1 cup of mango cubes
- ½ cup of lime juice

1. This recipe is about as straightforward as it gets, just takes your cup of water, mango cubes, and lime juice and put them in a blender.
2. Blend these ingredients, pour in a glass, and get ready to drink up.

75. Paleo Cookies

Even during the 30-Day Paleo Challenge, you could use a treat, and these Paleo Cookies are the best way to do it! Just mix, bake and serve up this batch of Paleo Cookie goodness!

Here are the exact ingredients:
- 1 cup chopped bananas
- ½ cup chopped apples
- ¼ cup of raw chopped walnuts
- ¼ cup of coconut milk
- ¼ cup of flax
- ¼ cup of cinnamon
- ¼ cup of baking soda
- ¼ cup of olive oil

1. Set your oven to 350 degrees.
2. Now take out a medium-sized mixing bowl and add your cup of chopped bananas, your ½ cup of chopped apples, and your ¼ cup of chopped walnuts.
3. Stir these ingredients together well before adding your ¼ cup of coconut milk, your ¼ cup of flax, your ¼ cup of cinnamon, and your ¼ cup of baking soda.
4. Stir all of these ingredients together well.
5. Now get out a cooking sheet and evenly coat it with your ¼ cup of olive oil. Now take your (clean) hands and use them to shape your cookies out of your dough in the mixing bowl.
6. Place these drops of mixture onto the cookie sheet.
7. Make sure that they are evenly spaced apart and then place your cooking sheet into the oven.
8. Let the cookies cool for about 15 minutes. These Paleo Cookies are done!

76. Sweet Paleo Potato Fries

If you need a pick-me-up, these Sweet Paleo Potato Fries will hit the spot! Treat yourself to some Sweet Paleo Potato Fries today!

Here are the exact ingredients:
- 1 cup chopped sweet potato
- One egg white
- ¼ cup of chili powder
- ¼ cup of garlic powder
- ¼ cup of onion powder

- ¼ cup of sat

1. Get out your sweet potatoes and peel them, before chopping them up and depositing them into a mixing bowl.
2. Now add your egg white and stir these ingredients together.
3. Add these ingredients to a medium-sized saucepan and add your ¼ cup of chili powder, your ¼ cup of garlic powder, your ¼ cup of onion powder, and your ¼ cup of salt.
4. Turn your burner off and serve when ready.

77. Apple Cherry Crumble Cake

This paleo dessert is a tasty treat at the end of the day! Save this recipe for when you need it!

Here are the exact ingredients:
- 1 cup of chopped cherries
- 1 bowl of chopped apples
- ¼ cup of lemon juice
- ¼ cup of cashews
- ¼ cup of cinnamon
- ¼ cup of coconut oil

1. Set your oven to 350 degrees. Now take your cup of chopped cherries, your cup of chopped apples and put them in an oven-safe dish.

2. Now get out a small mixing bowl and add your ¼ cup of lemon juice, your ¼ cup of cashews, your ¼ cup of cinnamon, and your ¼ cup of coconut oil.
3. Mix these ingredients well and then pour them over your apples and cherries in the dish.
4. Place your bowl in the oven and allow it to cook for about a half hour.
5. Once your half hour has passed, turn off your oven and let the Apple Cherry Crumble Cake to cool.

78. Paleolithic Lemon Soufflé

This recipe allows you to make a side dish with some real class! Paleolithic Lemon Soufflé is an excellent reward for your 30-Day Paleo Challenge!

Here are the exact ingredients:
- ½ cup of lemon juice
- 1 scooped out the lemon rind
- 1 cup of coconut milk
- ¼ cup of honey
- Three eggs

1. Set your oven to 350 degrees.
2. Now get out a medium-sized mixing bowl and add your ¼ cup of lemon juice, your ¼ cup of honey, your three eggs, and your coconut milk.
3. Mix these until they constitute one fine paste.

4. Now take your scooped-out lemon rind and put it in the center of a lightly greased cooking sheet.
5. Pour your ingredients into the lemon rind.
6. Now place the cooking sheet in the oven and allow it to cook for about 15 minutes until the soufflé rises.
7. Your Paleolithic Lemon Soufflé is now ready for business.

79. Paleo Pocket Popsicles

With its excellent taste and its close adherence to the guidelines of the 30-Day Paleo Challenge, this recipe is a real delight! Paleo Pocket Popsicles are easy to make and even more straightforward to eat!

Here are the exact ingredients:
- 4 cups of coconut water
- ½ cup of lime juice
- ¼ cup of lime zest
- 1 cup chopped raspberries
- 1 bowl of chopped peaches
- 1 cup of coconut milk
- ½ cup of lemon juice
- 1 cup of chopped blueberries

1. Take 12 Dixie cups and put them on a cooking sheet.
2. Now mix your ingredients in a mixing bowl and deposit the mixture into each of the Dixie cups.
3. Now stick a straw in the center of each one of the batters.

4. Place in the freezer and allow to freeze over the next few hours. You can now go ahead and pocket these popsicles!

80. Banana Pudding

With recipes like this, the 30-Day Paleo Challenge isn't a challenge at all! This banana pudding is hands down the best paleo friendly pudding in town!

Here are the exact ingredients:
- 1 cup of chopped banana
- ¼ cup of coconut milk
- ¼ cup of chia seeds
- ¼ cup of vanilla extract

1. Add your cup of chopped banana and your ¼ cup of coconut milk to a blender shut the lid, and thoroughly blend.
2. Next, take the cap off and add your ¼ cup of chia seeds to the mix.
3. Shut the top again, and pulse the blender a few more times just to mix the seeds into the rest of the ingredients.
4. Now transfer the contents of your blender to a mixing bowl and add your ¼ cup of vanilla extract.
5. Stir all of these ingredients together well.
6. Put a lid on the mixing bowl and place it in the fridge to settle.

7. After about an hour or so, take out of the refrigerator and serve.

Chapter 7: Tips to Help You Meet your Challenge

Get Enough Exercise

No matter what your diet is, the power of exercise cannot be underestimated. And if you think about it, our Paleolithic Ancestors were a pretty active bunch. They walked several miles a day, were able to outrun wooly mammoths, swam lakes, rivers, and streams looking for fish and climbed trees to get fruit, so we know that they got their exercise! So, having that said, practice is part and parcel of the paleo challenge.

And although you don't have to outrun a wooly mammoth, you should be able to do some cardio vascular exercise—whether it is going for a walk or just running in place in your own home. All of these exercises are enough to get your heart pumping and improve your circulation. You should also invest in some upper body strength training such as push-ups, pull-ups, or weightlifting. If you get enough exercise, your 60-day paleo challenge will be a breeze!

Take the Challenge with a Friend

Everything is just a little bit easier when we have a partner to experience challenge with. And the same goes for the Paleo challenge. If you have a friend or significant other who is interested in changing their diet, you should encourage them to partake in the 30-day paleo challenge right along with you.

That way you can have a constant source of encouragement, even as you help each other along. Besides—that's how our Paleolithic ancestors lived out their lives in the first place. They lived and worked as a team in their efforts to hunt and gather and you can your personal friend and ally can also work together to complete your 30-day paleo challenge successfully.

Allow yourself to be Hungry

Hunger is normal. And experiencing hunger in between meals is just part of the metabolic process of your body as it uses up its nutrient resources during a day. Your desire is just a side effect of this process that alerts you to what your body needs to have replenished. Allow yourself to be hungry, so you can witness this mechanism at work.

Get Fresh Air and Sunshine

Our paleo ancestors spent almost all of their time outside. This is where they got their bread and butter through hunting, foraging, and gathering. But today for most of us the reverse is true, for most of us, we spend the majority of our time inside. But we are not so far removed from the paleolithic past that we can't still benefit a great deal from getting a little bit of fresh air and sunshine.

Sunshine itself has been proven beneficial to the human body in the form of the Vitamin D that it bombards us with. Vitamin D helps the body in a wide variety of ways; including the development of bones. So, 30-day paleo challenge or not, in the long run, merely getting some fresh air and sunshine can help you out tremendously.

Get some Sleep

Sleep is an essential component of how our body's function and most especially how they metabolize and process the foods that we eat. If you are not getting enough sleep, your body will not be able to efficiently take in all of the nutrients you are feeding it. To get your body running and humming like a well-oiled machine, you are going to have to get some sleep!

Track Your Progress

As you continue on the Paleo diet, you need to be as patient as possible as you monitor your progress. Keep track of the small things, and take note of milestones along the way. The Paleo Challenge is more of a marathon than it is a sprint. So be patient and take stock of what you have already accomplished. The more of your success that you see, the more it will encourage you to go forward.

Weight loss is the most apparent form of accomplishment of any diet, but perhaps you can monitor improvements in other areas of your life as well. Do you have less stress towards the end of your 30-day challenge? Do you feel happier? Are those around you begin to notice a definite shift in direction in your general attitude? These are all potential benefits of the 30-day challenge and well worth nothing as you track your progress.

Experiment with Organs

No, this section is not advising you to become a doctor and analysis with organ transplants! Because when we say "experiment with organs" as it pertains to Paleo means experimenting with organ meats from animals. Although most of us nowadays strictly eat the muscle tissues of livestock, our ancestors got a large part of their nutrition through the consumption of organs such as the hearts, livers, and even lungs, of the animals that they hunted.

Even if you initially turn your nose at the thought, just consider the fact that organ meat from a cow doesn't taste that much different from other beef consumed from the cow's body. Beef hearts feel reasonably similar to other kinds of beef, so don't be afraid to experiment. Organs are no doubt the healthiest part of an animal to consume. They are loaded with vitamins and minerals that you can't get any other way. Our paleolithic ancestors loved to eat them, and you should too!

Eat Your Leftover Food

Leftovers get a bad rap, but the truth is, they can save you a whole lot of time, energy, and stress! If you have any extra food for lunch that you don't feel like eating, because you are full or pressed for time, don't throw it away. Instead, put it in a plastic container and save it for later, that way you can have some fully prepped food ready for you by the time the next day comes around again!

Have a Hobby

We all have hobbies that we gain fulfillment from, but eating should not be one of them! If your hobby is staring at the TV and munching on a big old bag of potato chips, we need to correct that part of your routine! You should have plenty of fulfilling hobbies that have nothing at all to do with food in which you can invest your time. That way you will be more likely to eat only when you need nourishment and not just for something to do.

For our Paleolithic ancestors, after all, there was no such thing as eating out of boredom, they only ate to survive. For paleo man, his downtime was filled with non-food eating activity such as singing, storytelling, cave painting and the like. So, let's go back to those paleo days of yore and find ways to fulfill ourselves without continually filling our bellies. Find a good hobby.

Become a Good Cook

As this book demonstrates, eating the right foods is only one aspect of a successfully 30-day paleo challenge, since most of the recipes presented in this book require some essential preparation, you need to be a good cook as well. If you have never cooked much in your life, this book is a significant first step for you since the recipes presented here are all relatively straightforward, "no frills" and right to the point. Use this book as a stepping stone in your culinary career, and you will indeed become a good cook by the time your 30-day paleo challenge comes to a close.

Drink a Lot of water

Because our bodies are made up of 98% water, it is no wonder that we need to have replenishments of this resource on a daily basis. In fact, without new additions of water at least every three days, our bodies are unable to continue carrying out their functions. Digestion grinds to a halt without adequate H2O to facilitate the process, and our very hearts can't beat as they become water depleted. As you can see, this chemical combination called H2O is crucial, so make sure that you drink a lot of it!

Get a Handle on Your Caffeine Intake

As much as we love the smell of that coffee in the morning or perhaps the sudden rush of an energy drink in the evening. We need to get a handle on our caffeine intake. While caffeine in itself is not necessarily harmful to your results on the Paleo Challenge. If you can't even get through the day without downing three energy drinks, this is a problem that needs to be created, and by forcing your body to reboot and reprogram itself by going 30 days without continually consuming caffeine, you could much benefit in the process.

Quit Smoking

By most accounts, our Paleolithic Ancestors did not puff on cigars, cigarettes or hookahs, so to correctly simulate the conditions of their Paleolithic past, you shouldn't either. Smoking will only slow you down. There are so many toxic ingredients in cigarette smoke it will make your head spin. Many smokes because they think that it will help them lose weight.

They see the act of cigarette smoking as an act of negating their cravings for food. But quitting smoking right as you start the paleo challenge is an excellent tactic because it allows you to end one habit and replace it with another. So, for your health and future success, you may want to make yourself quit the smoking habit.

Don't Trust the Big-Name Food Companies

I know we like to believe everything we read on the back of a box, but the so-called "Nutrition Facts" derived from our processed food containers are not always being entirely truthful with us. We need to do some of our research. Don't place all of your faith in marketers and advertisers who merely wish for you to spend money. These organizations, after all, are the same ones that brought us harmful things such as high fructose, GMO's and trans-fat. Don't trust the big-name food companies. And if you think you don't need it; <u>they don't eat it.</u>

Use Mindful Eating to Help You Meet Your Goals

It is incredible how much we can benefit by merely practicing a little bit of mindfulness and being aware of where we are and what we are doing when we eat. Instead of thinking about the bills or the pressures at work, we need to focus on the food we are eating. We need to focus on the right here, and the power now. It may sound a little silly at first, but don't let your mind wander and allow yourself to focus on the act of eating itself. That way you can use mindful eating to help you meet your goals.

Conclusion

Thank you for reading this book.

I hope this book was able to help you to follow the paleo plan, eat only when you are hungry, and make sure that your foods contain lean meats, healthy fats, and a great variety of vegetables, for rapid weight loss good healthy.

The next step is to start your 60 day paleo diet challenge and take control of your life! The paleo diet will lead you to a healthier, happier life.